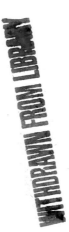

W9-DGN-172

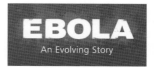

EBOLA

An Evolving Story

EBOLA
An Evolving Story

JAMES LYONS-WEILER

Ebola Rapid Assay Development Consortium, USA

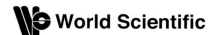 **World Scientific**

NEW JERSEY · LONDON · SINGAPORE · BEIJING · SHANGHAI · HONG KONG · TAIPEI · CHENNAI

2830376   MAR 1 5 2016

Published by

World Scientific Publishing Co. Pte. Ltd.

5 Toh Tuck Link, Singapore 596224

USA office: 27 Warren Street, Suite 401-402, Hackensack, NJ 07601

UK office: 57 Shelton Street, Covent Garden, London WC2H 9HE

Library of Congress Cataloging-in-Publication Data
Lyons-Weiler, James, author.
 Ebola : an evolving story / James Lyons-Weiler.
  p. ; cm.
 Includes bibliographical references and index.
 ISBN 978-9814675918 (hardcover : alk. paper) -- ISBN 9814675911 (hardcover : alk. paper) --
 ISBN 978-9814675925 (pbk. : alk. paper) -- ISBN 981467592X (pbk. : alk. paper)
 I. Title.
 [DNLM: 1. Hemorrhagic Fever, Ebola. 2. Ebolavirus. WC 534]
 RC140.5 . L96 2015
 616.9'2--dc23
                          2015013805

British Library Cataloguing-in-Publication Data
A catalogue record for this book is available from the British Library.

Printed by FuIsland Offset Printing (S) Pte Ltd Singapore

For Katiada

"Failure to discover air-borne infection... [doesn't] prove its absence."
— William Wells, 1934

"In our lifetimes, or our children's lifetimes, we will face a broad array of dangerous emerging 21st-century diseases, man-made or natural, brand-new or old, newly resistant to our current vaccines and antiviral drugs. You can bet on it."
— Dr. Lawrence Brilliant

"We must not be complacent. This is an unforgiving virus."
— Dr. Margaret Chan, WHO Director-General

"Progress is painfully slow. The virus is operating on virus time, and all the rest of us are operating on bureaucracy time. And the virus is winning, hands down."
— Dr. Michael Osterholm

The Truth always matters in Science.

Sources:

Brilliant L. The Age of Pandemics. *The Wall Street Journal.* May 2, 2009. [http://online.wsj.com/article/SB124121965740478983.html accessed Nov 29, 2014]

Wells WF. (1934) On air-borne infection: study II. Droplets and droplet nuclei. *Am J Hyg* **20:** 611–18.

About the Author

James Lyons-Weiler, PhD, lives in the wonderful township of Allison Park, PA, just north of Pittsburgh. He is a former AP Sloan Foundation postdoctoral fellow and evolutionary biologist with a background in evolutionary theory, molecular evolution, genetics, phylogenetics, biogeography, ecology, genomics, proteomics, bio-informatics, and clinical research. After conducting research in lowland Amazonia and in the high deserts of the Great Basin in the US Intermountain West, he has spent 16 years working in biomedical research with over 100 clinical researchers on a bewildering diversity of studies. He is the managing director of the Ebola Rapid Assay Consortium, focused on engineering better ways to detect *Ebolavirus* earlier. He is the proud father of two boys.

Preface

This is a book about humanity's intrinsic capacity to adapt in the face of crisis, examined from all perspectives: biological, psychological, sociological, and political. It is a condensation of everything I've learned about what we know, and what we do not know, about the strain of the *Ebolavirus* behind the 2014 outbreak. In the broadest sense, it is a call for a new era in progressive science. It is also a call for institutional reform, and an appeal for a broader appreciation of the importance of using what we have, stating clearly the limits of our knowledge, for the consistent use of logic and self-examined thinking in the face of a crisis, and in our everyday lives. It provides a framework, I hope, for necessary, open, in-depth discussions about the science of infectious diseases, like *ebolavirus* diseases, and the effects that the practices of society and our institutions have on our ability to adapt to the challenges that face us.

I have always admired ardent advocates for meaningful, objective scientific research. I have a deep philosophically rooted position on the value of science based on the idea that good science, whether basic or applied, should not be a waste of time for any of its stakeholders. Any book that touches on science should be held to this standard, including this one. Ideally, scientific books should be unbiased. This book is biased, and therefore, it is not meant to be a scientific treatise on Ebola. Rather, it is meant to be a reasoned and objective inquiry into what we know, and do not know, and to provide insights into flaws in our institutions and their charters.

It is in this spirit that I offer the facts, and interpretations of the significance of some of those facts, and the informed speculations, that appear in this book. It was also written with a deep sense of moral responsibility for the well-being of others, with little or no regard for the effects of its publication on my career as a scientist, for better or for worse. I wrote this book because I realized that it had to be written. It was written in part to relieve myself of the frustration of the obvious gaps in the logical processes involved in the fight to defeat Ebola. It is prescriptive in places, but without, I hope, any sense of hubris. It was written to help me sort out the barrage of seemingly conflicting information presented during the late summer/early autumn of 2014, which some have come to call the "Ebola in the US hysteria." Was it hysteria? Or were we woefully unprepared, ill-informed, and ill-advised? Were people correct to express concern, and fear? Interest in Ebola peaked in October, and fell precipitously in November. But the disease had only begun its ravages.

While I have participated in hundreds of studies in biomedical research, including some studies of viral infection, I am not a virologist. I am not in the field risking exposure. I do not treat patients. I do not study the ebolavirus in a BSL-4 level laboratory. I am not an epidemiologist trained in shutting down outbreaks, nor do I conduct contact tracing. In this sense, the argument could be made that I am not the right person to write this book.

In another sense, my personal background and my broad professional training and involvement in so many biomedical studies from an genomics, proteomics, genetics and bioinformatics perspective, combined with my deep training in the principles of ecology and evolutionary biology and my personal investment in the quality of science, perhaps place me in suitable position to ask the right questions, to identify key pieces of information in the published literature that, when brought together on one page, tell perhaps a different story about the biology of this strain of Ebola than the story we have been told. I read these papers with insights in molecular biology, ecology, evolutionary theory, population genetics, experimental design, biostatistics, genomics, and proteomics.

I helped create the field now known as "bioinformatics." I have worked on research studies from cell lines to animal models to clinical studies in diseases across the board. I am a believer in collaborative research, and I am an outside-of-the-box thinker. In fact, one might say that my mantra is: "There is no box." As my undergraduate genetics professor advertised, and as many of my colleagues will attest, I like to "question authority."

For this project, however, I have taken a cold, detached and sober scientific look at this crisis. Consider the testimony of Dr. Kent Brantly, EVD survivor and former medical director, Samaritan's Purse, to the Senate Health and Appropriations Committee and Health, Education, Labor and Pensions Committee on Sept 16, 2014:

> *Many have used the analogy of a fire burning out of control to describe this unprecedented Ebola outbreak. Indeed it is a fire — a fire straight from the pit of hell. We cannot fool ourselves into thinking that the vast moat of the Atlantic Ocean will keep the flames away from our shores. Instead, we must mobilize the resources needed to keep entire nations from being reduced to ashes.*

If you know of the suffering in Africa, you know there is never enough raw emotion. But this project demanded hard logic. From the WHO reports, I have been able to track the progress of the disease from when there were fewer than 100 cases to the present, with more than 25,500 cases and nearly 10,500 deaths. My analyses reveal a need for specific additions to approaches to medical treatment of EVD and the care of EVD patients. Specifically, given the data others have published, and that which I have compiled, it seems that we should not expect this disease to mostly involve hemorrhaging. Rather, hospitals around the world preparing for EVD cases should be prepared, contrary to expectations, to be able to disinfect and dispose of massive volumes of highly contagious vomit and feces; the optimal re-hydration may be less than supposed due to the increased likelihood of transmission with increased fluid intake.

My overall analysis of the symptomological reports and published data informs me that the shift in frequency and vomiting without prior warning is, possibly, a newly acquired mode of transmission: The incidence of vomiting is up, but the incidence of abdominal pain is down compared to past outbreaks. It is fair to speculate whether any of the mutations observed in the 2014 epidemic strain are causal of this new phenotype. Consider that one of the first records of concern over increased volumes of liquid waste that I encountered in the media was on Jan 3, 2015, in the *Boston Globe* article "Ebola response shows flaws in US system":

> *Dr. Paul Biddinger, Mass. General's chief of emergency preparedness, said hospitals did not understand "how different this disease was," producing liters upon liters of highly infectious fluid.*

Pair this with the initial firm conviction in the statements of US policy makers of the "facts" that *"We know this virus,"* and *"There are no mutations,"* and *"We are ready to handle Ebola cases in the US"*; it is also fair to say that in the CDC's need to reassure the public, they and our medical community may have, unwittingly, caused people around the world to consider dealing with this outbreak a task much easier than it actually was, and is.

My analysis also tells me that any meaningful response to outbreaks in the future will require immediate, thorough contact tracing, education in areas where the virus is likely to spread, and that we need to focus on developing vaccines and effective treatments and widely available home protection units. However, equally important to "bending the curve" to prevent outbreaks from becoming epidemics or pandemics will be building isolated treatment units and the development of diagnostic kits for ebolavirus that can detect the virus in asymptomatic infected persons to allow isolation and treatment before they become increasingly contagious. This is a mathematical factor, not a political or economic factor. It is in the interest of the public health to make treatment of EVD unnecessary. We need to be as adaptive as the virus: In these technologies, we need to anticipate that changes in the gene and protein sequences may influence the sensitivity and specificity of these tests, as well as the virulence and transmissibility of the disease. Finally, my analysis also points to a multifaceted needs for rapid assessment and re-evaluation of statements made by public health officials, and the public health practices and policies — conducted by the policy makers themselves — if we are going to succeed in shutting down this epidemic. The public deserves to know the worst case possibility, and its likelihood of occurrence.

I have always seemed to have had a knack for identifying key problems at any given time in my career. Perhaps I am simply drawn to solve hard problems. I have similarly been able to see efficient and elegant solutions to problems nearly instantly when given sufficient information about complex problems. These abilities have been both a blessing and curse. They have afforded me my career to date, in service of biological, clinical and translational research, as a bioinformatician. However they have also, at times cost me friends and professional relationships, as I have offered simple and elegant solutions to complex problems that have apparently flummoxed and stymied my colleagues for some time. I have been told, in nearly every professional position I have held, that I need to "slow down." I can only attribute this to the fact that my abilities, which I consider affording me special insight, are made limiting with a unique two-fold problem: First, I have often found it necessary to nearly reverse engineer my own solutions, and second, because while the solution itself seems self-evident, translating the solution and communicating it in terms that reveal an appropriate, step-wise logic, can be a much more arduous task. Simply seeing the solution has never been enough; sharing it in sufficient detail to convince the skeptic, or those concerned with preserving the status quo, has often proven itself to be the most arduous part. In part this is because I often find that significant gains in understanding are only possible by systematically challenging foundational thinking. I most find myself wondering what we could learn by systematically altering the assumptions that either make up, or are derived from, the background knowledge upon which we base a given scientific query. In this sense, I am a devout deconstructionist;

however, this is done solely to determine whether gains in understanding can be made so we are ready for them when new findings become available that challenge our old assumptions. The history of science is laden with things we used to "know," so it seems sensible to challenge old assumptions and see what logically follows. This approach to science is rarely conducted, and is rarely encouraged; young scientists are encouraged instead to add new leaves to the tree of knowledge, to build on what is known, not shake the tree's trunk, or better, pull it up by its roots.

This is apparently what has happened with my understanding of the social dynamics in the response to the threat of Ebola. During the summer of 2014, I could see a pattern. Early on I wondered where the calls for funding for Ebola were in the national media. I could see this outbreak was larger, and spreading faster, than those I had paid attention to in the past. I recognized a series of specific limitations of existing medical, epidemiological, sociological and cultural assumptions in terms of assertions, some of which were mere assumptions, made about the current strain. Many of these on the face of it appeared to not be correct to me, and certainly not warranted by data readily available to those who know how to access it. I saw interpretations of causal factors in the spread of the disease in African offered, and accepted as fact, without clear validation, while other, more biological factors were overlooked or minimized. I saw errors in terms of the clinical interpretation of the outcome of existing tests for Ebola (i.e., incorrect interpretation of negative results prior to 21 days); I witnessed misrepresentation of facts published in major medical research journals, and in sworn testimony to Congress; I saw individuals willing to overlook their own use of fear as a basis for policy that could affect millions, all the while insisting that we should never base policies on fear. I saw people for one reason, or the other, making decisions and indeed behaving in ways for their own self-monitoring that they themselves would not recommend for others in their exact situation. I saw the press in the US agree to a White House request to restrict the amount of information they publish about suspected cases of

EVD in the US. And I saw, and still see, the world's population at risk due to the first true EVD epidemic in history, when the clues that suggest the need for a different approach may in fact be found in the best place for them to hide: In plain sight.

I have worked hard to connect the points from beginning to end in my renderings of the problems, and the proposed solutions. Not all of the solutions proposed are mine, however, any errors are my own. Where I have failed, I apologize. I leave it to the reader, and, eventually, good scientific research, to determine whether any of my informed speculations (hypotheses) are well-founded. Given the gravity of the situation, they are worth considering — as soon as possible. Even as I was writing this book, events seemed to provide data that contradicted public statements, and increased my suspicions that we were both medically, scientifically, and politically off track. In the final chapter, I offer a rational analysis of decision making and thinking in a form of cost–benefit analysis that uses the same currency for rational and irrational aspects of problem solving. My hope in offering this is that people in the right positions in high institutions of influence will use this method for an informal, private analysis of their own finite thinking, informally, or formally, to reveal in a purely rational manner to themselves the factors at play that may be causing them to hold onto to cherished notions. It may prove to be useful in other ways, such as conflict resolution. I hope so. I hope it can stimulate new ways of thinking and solving complex issues in society using a process within which people can learn to objectively discuss their own assumptions and conclusions, in which they can more easily consider whether they actually know what they think they know, and to help them think, as I like to refer to it as, in a "metacognitive" manner. Rational people change their minds in the face of new evidence. In the face of their own ignorance, rational people say: "I don't know."

Hopefully, in the future, we can receive robust and unapologetic "We don't know the answer to that question yet," rather than answers that someone might wish, and is hoping, are true. A rationale discourse, if you will.

I want to thank certain people, many of whom may be surprised to read their names in this list: Costas Maranas and Tong Li, who were among the first to take a step in the direction of moving toward a radical new approach to caring for EVD patients; Prof. Klaus Schulten, Boon Gong Chong and Kevin Plaxco, who continuously holds my hope, based on the fact that a solution must be found, to an appropriate empirical standard; Niki Lynn Page, and colleagues at the Penn State University's Strategic Interdisciplinary Research Office, for stepping up to the task of providing professional support in our fund-seeking effort to move the ultra-sensitive reactive matrix amplifier concept forward; Dr. Gavin MacGregor-Skinner, who stands apart from all others in my view as a voice of impassioned reason and infinite energy for educating and protecting the public; Dr. Michael Osterholm, whose presentation at Johns Hopkins should, in my view, be required viewing for all medical students; Ken Kam, for his vision in calling reform for simplifying compassionate use of novel drugs to treat the terminally ill and other people who might not wish to die on placebo; Dr. Erica Ollmann Saphire, for sharing key information regarding the epitopes in *ebolavirus* Gp1Gp2 protein with our consortium, and to the following people for inspiring me to be myself in all things: Dr. Peter Rosenbaum, Dr. Masatoshi Nei, Dr. Guy Hoelzer, and Dr. Robin Tausch, and the hundreds of investigators who have shared their research with me over the past seven years for giving me the chance to help them take their studies up a notch on objectivity with translational approaches towards positive clinical impact, especially Dr. Sandra Founds, Dr. Carol Feghali-Bostwick, Dr. John Kirkwood, and Dr. Stephen Dobrowolski, all who, in my view, provide excellent role models for new biomedical scientists. To Dr. Paul Colinvaux, who used to inspire my questioning of assumptions, thank you for your stories of how Dr. Dan Livingstone would say, if someone were to ever show one of his hypotheses wrong: *"Wouldn't that be wonderful!"* And to Dr. Olja Finn, for never giving up on progressive treatments for cancer, including the remarkable work on effective cancer vaccines. Thanks to Bob Banerjee for words of wisdom and for our chats and discussions.

Thanks to Brian Murtagh, who encouraged me to begin broadcasting these observations and ideas, and for pointing out that conservative politicians are, ironically, showing a sudden and extreme interested in the processes of evolution. Thank you to my friend and five-time cancer survivor, Dr. Andy von Eschenbach, who had the courage to challenge the NCI and those working with the NCI to actually seek a cure for cancer within five years. Your leadership inspired and sustained me more than you may know. Of course a huge thank you to Grace Innes for hearing all of my ideas out in their most nascent of stages, you carried me during my darkest times. Thank you Ben for your suggested edits, both technical and scientific, and thank you to Ben and Zach for our discussions, and for being two very important reasons for me wanting the medical and scientific community to get it right, for the right reasons. You have both provided infinite moral support during the weakest moments, and you make me extremely proud to say I am a father.

Just two month prior to this writing, the situation in Sierra Leone was deplorable; there discoveries of wards in hospitals cordoned off, with the dead piled high. In December 2014, Dr. Peter Kilmarx, CDC director for Zimbabwe, reported to *The New York Times* that patient care was being moved into the homes of the patients, and he used the word "defeat":

> *"For the clinicians it's admitting failure, but we are responding to the need," Dr. Kilmarx said. "There are hundreds of people with Ebola that we are not able to bring into a facility."*

Schools have been closed. Hospitals have been closed. Health care workers have gone on strike for the lack of resources needed to ensure their safety and to treat patients. Elections have been postponed. Entire towns have been quarantined — a technique not used in public health management since the middle ages. Thousands of children have been left orphaned, and even close relatives fear taking the children in. Christmas parties have been banned, and elections postponed. Travel and trade bans have been put into force. Bodies have literally been piled up, and in some places, people have crawled into the forest... to die. People are being buried in mass graves without identification. The proper treatment of other diseases, such as malaria, has been severely obstructed. Harvests have been canceled, and the peace dividends of the last 10 years — a growing economy, increasing literacy, and national infrastructure — are all being obliterated. While the cost in terms pain and suffering and of loss of peaceful human lifetime cannot be measured, the eventual financial costs, both direct and indirect, to Western African countries affected by EVD, is measured in the billions of dollars.

The research community, the medical community, and the public health community were caught off guard by this epidemic in many ways. We have not stockpiled immunoglobulins for passive immunotherapy, for example. In a recent discussion, Dr. Kyle Bibby, who studies the disposal of infectious agents, shared this sentiment:

> *We were caught unprepared. One thing we should learn from this epidemic: investment measures on critical research questions are needed before an outbreak.*

In conducting research for this book, certain themes emerged. These include:

— We were unprepared.
— We do not use all of the resources we have.
— Our institutions are too focused on control, and not sufficiently focused on facilitating solutions.
— We don't yet know what we need to know to end the epidemic.
— We do not know the full extent of the biological differences between the Ebola guinea strain and strains from past outbreaks, including the species *Zaire ebolavirus*.
— The virus may have acquired an enhanced ability for transmission via gastrointestinal effects.
— Certain important interpretations of available data expressed as public health policies are not logical and may help promote the spread of the virus.

— Indirect transmission may be more prevalent than expected from past strains.
— If EVD takes hold in a densely populated large metropolitan area, infectious waste inactivation and management alone will overwhelm any health care system in any country.
— The education of the public in areas at risk of EVD outbreaks should continue between outbreaks.
— The policies and practices of the FDA with respect to clinical trial has led to innumerable unreported deaths in patients who could have been, but were not treated, with novel promising drugs.

This book was written over the course of four months. Now, in February 2015, the outlook is neither dim, nor bleak, but it is quite sobering. We cannot let up. Resurgence of the disease is guaranteed; the goal at this time is to get to zero new patients and to prevent EVD from becoming endemic to our species. The American public should know that this epidemic had — retains the potential — to be utterly disastrous for Africa, and other parts of the world where poverty is endemic and population density is high. We must constantly work toward solutions of all kinds to bring the number of cases to zero.

This book is dedicated to the people in the front lines of this war against Ebola, especially the children like Katiada, who have lost their lives, or one or both parents, to people who have lost loved ones, and also optimistically to the good people of Earth in the year 2030, for they will include the survivors of the outbreak and their descendants. To honor the lives of those who have passed, we must be bold enough to admit our ignorance, and then to learn in earnest from our mistakes so future outbreaks are caught early, and future epidemics and pandemics are more readily prevented. It is through the admission of ignorance that we can begin to rationally formulate and prioritize important research questions.

Contents

1

Origins of the Epidemic

It began with the death of one little boy. His name was Emile, and he lived in a tiny village in forested Guinea called Meliandou.

His mother, Sia, tried to care for the boys as well as any mother would have, but she, too, soon fell ill, and died, with bleeding symptoms. Sia, who was pregnant, and her mother, were caring for Emile's sister Philomene, who died shortly thereafter with dark, bloody diarrhea and vomiting. Sia's mother died next, with symptoms similar to Philomene's. Two people who attended the grandmother's funeral returned to their village of Guéckédou, and infected a health care worker and their own family members. By February 2014, the virus had spread to Macenta, Nzérékoré, and Kissidougou.

No one knows how Emile contracted EVD in December. Perhaps he was fed some bushmeat, such as meat from a fruit bat. Some thought perhaps a vector of some kind, a tick, or a flea, injected the virus into his body. A report in December 2014 indicated that he had played under a tree that harbored an insectivorous bat species. Regardless of how he contracted it, no one in Emile's village of Meliandou could have suspected EVD. Their community resides deep in the forested area of Guinea, where many other culprits, such as cholera, typhoid, and Lassa fever, could have explained his symptoms. The infant death rate in Guinea is 10 times as high compared to that in the United States, and is especially high in the isolated areas, where there are few hospitals and doctors. The village is located near the nexus of a border with remote areas of two other countries: Sierra Leone and Liberia. Cross-border trade among locals in these countries is routine; the people in these remote areas in the three countries feel and share kinship regardless of national border, carrying the virus with them. For months, the virus spread through families and villages and borders traveling quickly on improved roads. As people fell ill, their family members cared for them. Sick children were carried by their parents; older children were moved to hospitals in wheelbarrows. The virus' aim was deadly, killing over 90% of its victims.

Four months later, in March, 2014, nearly 4,000 miles away, central processing units spinning electrons in computers at Children's Hospital in Boston picked up blips suggesting a "mystery hemorrhagic fever" in forested areas of southeastern Guinea. Nine days would pass before the WHO doctors could recognize the uptick in deaths, and finally sound the alarm: Ebola.

Four months had passed between Emile's death and the WHO announcement of an outbreak of Ebola. Four months is an unusually long incubation period for Ebola to be passed among locals without detection. In the past, outbreaks had typically been localized, with a high fatality rate, and they were recognizable in part due to hemorrhaging and a high mortality rate. The symptoms had been characteristic and increasing in severity: fever, aches, pains, vomiting, diarrhea, and then exhaustion, followed by body rash, and coma via loss of blood pressure shock. During the Sudan Ebola quasispecies outbreak in the Democratic Republic of the Congo, 76 people got sick, of whom 59 died. These outbreaks had, in the past, been recognizable in part due to hemorrhaging. High prevalence of typical tell-tale bleeding from eyes, ears, nose and mouth gave the disease its traditional name: "Ebola hemorrhagic fever" (EHF)." We know now that this occurred as a result of more and more cells producing more and more virus particles, especially white blood cells (Wauquier *et al.*, 2010), causing the immune system unleashes a last-ditch "cytokine storm," which itself does massive tissue damage. As the disease spread in early 2014, the doctors treating patients starting dying, and hospitals in the provincial towns of Guéckédou and Macenta (Fig. 1.1) may have been more

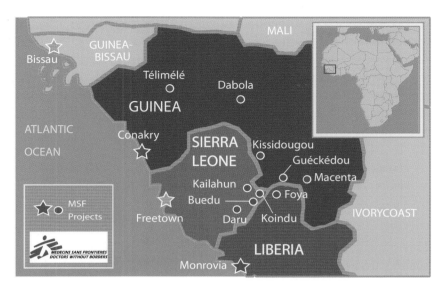

Fig. 1.1 Map of Western African countries at the center of the epidemic. Capital cities and Doctors Without Borders Project (MSF) sites are shown. "Ground Zero" village Meliandou, where Emile and his family lived at the onset of the 2013/2014 Ebola crisis, lies east of Guéckédou. Image credit: © 2014, MSF. Used with permission. http://www.msf.ca/en/article/ebola-west-africa-epidemic-out-control.

likely to correctly diagnose their patients, and themselves; however, somehow they, too missed the signs of Ebola. Perhaps they, too, considered cholera, malaria, or other types of fevers from the region with similar symptoms. It now seems that there was less bleeding.

Early in the outbreak, certainly no one in the region expected Ebola. No county in Western Africa had seen an outbreak of EVD. According to Dr. Margaret Chan, Director-General of the World Health Organization (WHO), the ecological conditions, the wildlife species (fauna), and hunting practices, that are ripe for a zoonotic transfer of *Ebolavirus* to humans exist in 22 African countries. So far, outbreaks had occurred in only five African countries: Democratic Republic of the Congo (Zaire), Uganda, Gabon, Sudan, and Ivory Coast.

Even if they had somehow known that this region was afflicted with EVD, their description of the emergence of EVD in West Africa would have included a key discrepancy in their observation from past outbreaks: While most patients suffered from fever, vomiting and severe diarrhea, fewer (~40%) suffered from visible hemorrhaging. Compared to the first EHF outbreak of the Sudan virus, in 1976:

> *Haemorrhagic manifestations were common (71%), being present in half of the recovered cases and in almost all the fatal cases.*

(WHO Bull, World Health Organization 1978; **56(2)**: 247–70)

This statistic is important, but is rarely referenced. The number of health care workers that were becoming infected was very high; by August, over 216 health care workers had died. Around 5% of all cases in this outbreak have been health care workers. This is in the context in some countries in which there are very few doctors. In Guinea, the country in which the epidemic began as an outbreak, there are only 0.1 doctors per 1,000 people; in Sierra Leone, 0.022; in Liberia, about 0.014 (WHO). In the US, there are about 2.5 doctors/1000 people. In fact the WHO reports that 45.8% of WHO member states report to have less than one physician per 1,000 people. The death rates among the infected were initially very high (>90%); these have tapered now to just >50%. The losses of health care workers represent the virus fighting back directly against the health care system, which in some of the poorest areas of these countries, is virtually non-existent. The virus attacks everything we throw at it: In December 2014 we learned that some UN peacekeepers had contracted EVD. Transmission is thus far understood to require direct contact of *Ebolavirus* with a mucous membrane, either in the eye, mouth, or nose. However, to understand transmission risks of an infectious agent, one must have an understanding of the biology of the virus.

Perhaps the single largest factor contributing the initial exponential spread of the virus remains: The international global response was deplorable. The urgency communicated by WHO officials and some at the UN has been described as frantic; they were literally screaming that no one understood the seriousness of this outbreak. Dr. Tom Frieden, Director of the CDC, was among the earliest voices with a clarion call to pay attention to this particular outbreak. The lag in the international response was not likely due to complacency; between outbreaks, the WHO and the CDC witness many false positive alarms for infectious disease outbreaks and, like cancer treatment, "watchful waiting" often *is* the standard protocol. It seems no protocol is in place to attempt to rapidly ground-truth each and every possible report. The WHO held an international meeting and concluded that a vaccine was desperately needed, as a first priority. The Obama administration's response to the pleas for help included plans for Domestic Preparedness and pledges of aid to Ebola-affected countries. This has included use of US troops to build hospitals. The international response has increased in response to the size and duration of the epidemic. In Jan 2015, China added 232 army medical workers to the 43 army doctors and 35 specialists from their CDC.

The most vocal critics of the US response to the crisis first came in the form of interrogation by Congressional Representatives in House Oversight hearings at the US Capitol. Over the course of a few days, the principle leaders of institutions in the US at the forefront of the outbreak — the CDC, the NIH, the NIAID, and Major General James Lariviere, deputy director of political-military affairs in Africa for the Defense Department, were questioned about everything from the nature of the threat to the misleading information provided by the CDC on their website. There was a mid-term election coming, and the air was thick with finger pointing and politicization of a grave topic. Senators were visibly agitated, and panelists were, at times, literally shaking.

DHS Inspector General John Roth testified that while the agencies in question had purchased antivirals and PPE, there was no fully developed understanding of what an epidemic of this sort would require, and no plans for who would receive what supplies.

Others testified that airport screening was not working. At the time, new cases of EVD were being announced even as the hearings proceeded.

Senator Chuck Grassley (IA) commented that he was "*scared to death of Ebola*," and later introduced a bill banning visas for people living in Ebola-affected countries. Congressional Representative Fred Upton (MI) asked CDC director Thomas Frieden why there was no fail-safe ban on people traveling from affected countries. Dr. Frieden's reply was that a ban would prevent them from tracing possible cases, to which Representative Fred Upton quipped: "*We should not let them in … period.*" Speaking with reporters after the hearings, Representative Cory Gardner (CO) took Dr. Frieden to task for his reasoning: "*That's like saying all children with chicken pox should stay in school so we know where they are.*" Representative Tim Murphy (PA) told news host Chris Wallace that he did not thinks "false assurances" were working. An epidemiologist, Dr. Vera F. Dolan, provided an affidavit citing the studies of experimental aerosol transmission in monkeys and suspected aerosol transmission in pigs as evidence for her support of enforced 21-day quarantine and travel restrictions. She wrote:

> *In my opinion, any individual who has visited the Ebola-affected African countries of Guinea, Sierra Leone, and Liberia should be quarantined for 21 days. Such individuals should be put on a "no-fly" list, to be kept in force until the officially declared end of the current Ebola epidemic.*

> — Mendocino County, CA, Court Affidavit, Oct 10, 2014

The NIH and the CDC have sought to reassure the American public that it is extremely unlikely that an epidemic of the type seen in Western African could happen in the US. They have confidence in our ability to identify any cases, and shut down any transmission chains. However, the experiences in the late summer and autumn of 2014 did anything but reassure many. The US did not seem ready.

In fact, we were not. Another sign of the CDC's lack of readiness for an epidemic of this scale is that the software for Ebola data collection was designed so only a single person could enter data at a time. The CDC was not quite ready to track people large numbers of people. The system was updated for multiple people to enter data; however, some wonder why the CDC is writing software in the first place. To guarantee state of the art data collection, companies like Apple and Microsoft could design apps and provide hardware that uses state of the art wireless technologies. This type of oversight in preparedness had led some to describe the US response as "clumsy" (Johnson, 2014).

Back in Western Africa, any and every bit of help in any form was then, and still is needed. In Sierra Leone, especially, it seems as of this writing, if every country and company gave all, it still might not be enough.

The Wee Beastie

Ebola is a terrifying monster. Its genome is devastatingly brilliant, seemingly designed like a monkey puzzle tree. Under the right terrifying conditions, it has the capacity to kill millions in a few months' time. While policy makers in the US ponder how wrong it would be to close our borders to reduce the risk of it spreading here, this virus has already closed borders in numerous African countries; it is waging war on their economies and the psyche of their peoples; it has brought the world media's attention and focus away from the threat of a third world war (the Ukraine crisis), and it shows no sign of stopping in spite of a massive, concerted international effort.

The human genome has some 47,000 known and suspected (predicted) genes.

This Thing has a mere seven protein-coding genes.

Genes translated into proteins in human cells are encoded by a simple alphabet of four letters: A, T, C, and G. Any combination of three of these letters encodes an encrypted word (codon), which, is then translated by special proteins in the cell (ribosomes) into a word (amino acid). The amino acids encoded in series by the letters in a gene can be thought of as a sentence that represents three levels of information about a protein: its primary sequence, and its secondary and tertiary (three-dimensional) structure. A protein's structure is thus determined in large part by its primary sequence of amino acids, which is in turn encoded by the string of four letters within the DNA sequence of the gene encoding the protein. Of the 47,000 genes in the human genome, some have overlapping reading frames (they encode more than one gene).

Like most viruses, the replication cycle and component assembly take place in the cytoplasm of infected cells. At first, the "body" is assembled as an "inclusion body," made up of ribonucleoprotein (RNP) complexes consisting of RNA and four nucleocapsid proteins: The nucleoprotein (NP), VP35, the polymerase (L), and VP30. Assembly begins with the virus hijacking the host genome, causing it to make viral RNA for the viral genes. The first structure that appears is a helix made of the NP gene RNA itself. This provides the core structure of the viral nucleocapsid. A gene called the matrix protein (VP40) transports nucleocapsids to the cell surface, where they bud off as virions (Noda *et al.*, 2006; Adu-Gyamfi *et al.*, 2014), a process facilitated by the matrix protein VP24 (Radzimanowski *et al.*, 2014). VP24 likely has many other functions, as it can associate with copies of itself in numerous configurations.

There are numerous unusual aspects of *Ebolavirus* biology. We do not yet know all of the functions of each gene. Many of *Ebolavirus'* genes share overlapping reading frames with its neighbors. That is, the beginning part of the protein-coding portion of some genes is encoded, in part, by the ending coding sequence of the gene located in front of them in the genome. This is unusual in molecular biology. A gene's 3′ (right end) sequence bleeds into the 5′ start of the next gene. The genes are transcribed serially, and replication stops after each gene (Muhlberger *et al.*, 1996). Transcription is re-started by the minor nucleoprotein, VP30 (Martinez *et al.*, 2008). Some of the genes have stretches of

Table 1.1   Names and Known Roles of the Genes in _Zaire ebolavirus_

1. Nucleoprotein (NP)	Provides the core structure of the viral nucleocapsid
2. Polymerase complex protein (VP35)	Inhibits virus infection-induced transcriptional activation of IFN regulatory factor 3 (IRF-3) responsive mammalian promoters
3. Matrix protein (VP40) ("Transformer")	Transports nucleocapsids to the cell surface for incorporation into virions
4. Virion spike glycoprotein precursor (GP)	Orchestrates host cell entry as Gp1Gp2 protein complex; immune system evasion
5. Minor nucleoprotein (VP30)	Re-initiates transcription between gene pauses
6. Membrane-associated protein (VP24)	Mediates virion budding off
7. RNA-dependent RNA polymerase (L)	Conducts viral RNA synthesis

nucleotide bases, or intergenic "spacer" sequences, between them. One intergenic region is 144 nucleotide bases in length. The functions of the intergenic sequences are largely unknown (Brauberger *et al.*, 2014), but may play a role in re-initiation of transcription between genes.

One of the genes (GP for "glycoprotein") actually encodes two proteins transcribed from the same gene that work in concert to enact host cell penetration. The source of the difference between the two proteins encoded by one gene is ribosomal slippage, caused by a short series of repeated nucleotide bases, specifically "AAAA" (adenines), within the gene's protein-encoding sequence. The first protein, Gp1, acts as a sort of doorman, opening the host cell membrane while its sister protein, Gp2, shoots a grenade — a copy of the RNA genome — into the cell, allowing a virion entry. These two proteins are the focus of most research on a vaccine for

Ebolavirus. After the virus penetrates the host cell, it initiates production of proteins toward making more virions. It goes about replicating as many copies of itself as possible, hijacking the protein production resources in the cell (like most viruses do). This virus, however, is both terribly infectious (a small dose is sufficient to take hold in a person), and virulent (lethal). The host genome produces so many copies of the messenger RNA for the proteins needed by the virus, and the host cell's ribosomes work overtime to produce so many copies of the proteins from the messenger RNAs (mRNAs), that the host cell then secretes *Ebolavirus* in the space between cells. Thus new virions are born, ready to infect more cells.

The Molecular Battlefield

Among the first priorities in any effective battle plan is to weaken the defenses, and this is just what Ebola does. It attacks critical cells that are part of the immune system. In fact, it conscripts these cells for its own purposes by making them produce more virions. First, Ebola attacks the first responder white blood cells (neutrophils). The patient experiences flu-like symptoms, general pain, and tiredness. After a few days, they may find themselves with gastrointestinal distress, with either bloody vomit or diarrhea. Clinically, they will be found to have abnormal white blood cell counts: High neutrophils and low lymphocytes. The virus finds its way to the large white blood cells (macrophages), causing the release of cytokines. Cytokines are proteins that mediate cell–cell signals, like an SOS. However, a positive feedback loop results from *Ebolavirus* infections, leading to prolonged, intense inflammation that does not help. The liver is then damaged, which causes system-wide problems with coagulation. Coagulation affects more than just blood; it is also a critical, ongoing process that helps maintain proper blood vessel integrity. Once the virus reaches the internal lining of small blood vessels, they lose their ability to hold blood, and system-wide hemorrhaging can occur. Patients enter shock due to low blood pressure, leading to coma, and death (Sullivan *et al.*, 2003).

As the disease progresses, Ebola unleashes a torrent of attacks, with progressive severity, on nearly all of the cells of the body. Cell type by cell type, the body becomes a virus-producing machine. Many signals between cell types become disrupted, or confused. To say this virus is ingenious is an understatement. The proteins of *Ebolavirus* have been likened to being shape-shifting "Transformers" (Bornholdt *et al.*, 2013). At different stages of the virus host cell infection/host cell obliteration cycle, one protein (VP40) protein morphs into three different shapes: A butterfly, a ring, and a linear shape, and each shape performs a different function, each critical to the propagation of the virus.

We know that people who fail to mount a sufficiently strong immune response to *Ebolavirus* tend to die. Our humoral immune system has numerous layers of defense, including the adaptive production of antibodies, the manufacturing of complement proteins, and the production of antimicrobial peptides. It reacts to foreign things (antigens) in our bodies by mounting a manifold attack. This attack, like any battle plan, takes time. The most important of these details is the enemy's identity, and our immune systems learn the identity of foreign molecules via adaptive learning. Our defenses against antigens are equally ingenious. The major histocompatibility complex gene system is one of the most complex gene expression systems known. A variety of copies of mRNAs are produced, and then jumbled via recombination to produce a wide diversity of possible peptides. These peptides may, by chance, fit the antigen shape to a greater or lesser extent. Adaptive immunity is enabled via the differential survival and production of antibodies with increasing match to antigens. It is a process of trial and error, followed by selection and feedback for the production of more of those combinations with the best fit to the antigen. The foreign antigens are targeted, and once targeted for destruction by white blood cells, they are (hopefully) engulfed, digested, and removed from the blood stream and interstitial fluids.

Our immune system also needs to be "smart" enough to adapt in a manner that allows it to avoid friendly fire. It needs to know self from non-self. This is achieved by constant readiness and drilling by the immune system: It retains sufficient ability to discriminate native proteins from foreign invaders only if it learns and re-learns self from non-self on a constant basis.

In this case, the foreign proteins in the virus are usually new to the host, and are, initially, invisible to immune surveillance. They easily infect macrophages (white blood cells), and may be in fact be carried around the body as these cell conduct surveillance. Many of Ebola's genes serve dual functions that aid in escaping immune surveillance. The membrane-associated protein VP24 delays the production of the immune system's interferons (IFNs) and IFN signaling (Leung *et al.*, 2006). Remarkably, it also folds into a pyramidal structure that binds STAT1 directly (Zhang *et al.*, 2012). Polymerase complex protein VP35 can cap double-stranded RNA (Cárdenas *et al.*, 2006), and interacts with IRF7 to prevent detection of the virus by immune cells (Audet and Kobinger, 2014). In addition to serving as the doorman for host cell entry, the GP1GP2 protein itself may further "moonlight" by actively folding to hide its most immunoreactive sites among it folds, or among cell-surface proteins (Cook and Lee, 2013).

As part of its battle plan, this hideous creature also causes cells in the body to overproduce and release a special protein that is not incorporated into the virion, but is instead found in high abundance in the interstitial areas between cells. This protein is called sGP. sGP is actually a partial sequence, or epitope, of the GP1 protein, and it plays a stealthy role that increases the odds of the virus' survival. sGP is produced in high quantities via an unusual mechanism: Gp1Gp2 transcription, like its translation, is imperfect; it stutters. About 80% of the transcripts of Gp1Gp2 are truncated, whereas 20% are edited to completion after translation. sGP seems to elicit a host immune response of its own, and it may, when the virus infects neutrophils, play a role in making them ineffective. This 80:20 ratio in favor of sGP works effectively to overwhelm and confound the immune system; antibodies specific to Gp1Gp2 will attack sGP preferentially, and while antibodies specific to Gp1Gp2 are also represented in the repertoire of the human adaptive immune response, sGP is produced in such great quantities that it effectively acts like flak, misleading the immune's guidance system away from the more relevant target, which of course is the Gp1Gp2 proteins on the virion coat itself. Remarkably, the GP gene also produces two additional proteins, namely sGP (Mehedi *et al.*, 2011) and Δ-peptide, a cleaved fragment (Volchkova *et al.*, 1999).

The structures of *Ebolavirus* proteins are of fundamental and key importance to humanity's counter-attacks on the virus. "The structural images of *Ebolavirus*," said Dr. Erica Ollman-Saphire in a Scripps Research Institute press release, "are like enemy reconnaissance. They tell us exactly where to target antibodies or drugs." Erica is a world-renowned leader in structural virology, with a strong background in ecology and evolutionary biology. It was her team that solved the structure of the Gp1Gp2 complex bound to a human antibody from a survivor. She knows first-hand the importance of evolutionary differences in *Ebolavirus* vaccine targets, and their potential effect on methods of diagnostics. As a viral amino acid sequence changes, it has the potential to change the viral protein's 3-D structure. Diagnostic kits such as ELISA and immunofluoresent assays depend on a good match between the antibodies used in the kit, and the sequence of the infectious agent. Without a good match, you're effectively shooting in the dark for diagnostics. Ebola is evolving fast; assays may miss a large number of cases if they are not updated to keep up with the virus. With vaccines, the same is true. In a recent press conference, CDC director Thomas Frieden revealed that the 2014/2015 vaccine for influenza was targeted primarily a less severe strain of H3N2 but is expected to be much less effective than expected, because another, "mutated," "Type A" strain is being found in about 90% of the clinical cases of influenza. As limited at the vaccine may be, it's still important for people to get their flu shots: The protection against H3N2 is still valuable, and even mismatched vaccines may still lessen the severity of the symptoms. In the new era of Ebola, there is a much added benefit to effective influenza vaccines: If more people are vaccinated, there will be fewer cases of possible EVD to triage in a future outbreak.

The studies of genetic variants in Ebola guinea are fascinating. In *Science* magazine, Gire *et al.* (2014) showed (a) Two to four times more nucleotide substitutions in Ebola guinea compared to previous outbreaks; and (b) larger numbers of non-synonymous (amino-acid changing) substitutions than in past outbreaks — consistent with expanding viral population size and purifying selection by the new host (us). They point to an interesting nucleotide substitution at a position in the RNA sequence for a gene encoding an editing site in the GP protein; could Ebola guinea have found another way to shape-shift? Has it acquired any new functions?

So far I have referred to Ebola as a Beastie, a Thing, and a Monster, and Erica likens its ability to shape-shift its proteins for different functions to that of a Transformer. We know diseases mostly by their symptoms. These are well documented in Ebola, but they are worth a very close look. Viruses depend on transmission to new hosts to survive. Due to graphic descriptions in Richard Preston's book *Outbreak*, many people will be familiar with the end-stage symptom, in which the virus begins to have an effect on the blood vessels, causing them to become porous (vascular leak). This can lead to bleeding from the eyes, ears, nose, and mouth. Organs in the body cease to function as they lose vascular integrity, and leak. At the latest stages, the patient is highly contagious, oozing millions of copies of the virus in every milliliter (a cube of fluid 1 cm × 1 cm × 1 cm). The body can remain infectious for weeks.

Stephen King called Richard Preston's description of the virus "one of the most horrifying things I've read in my whole life" (Random House/Preston). But this virus is no thriller. It's not an invisible character in a book, or movie, wantonly and senselessly killing. It is real, and it is horrifying to contemplate the devastation Ebola is wreaking on countries at the epicenter of the outbreak: Guinea, Sierra Leone and Liberia. It is tearing apart their population, their economy, and their institutions, including their health care systems. The destruction of societal infrastructure by EVD is geographically acute, and it also serves to multiply the infection rate. This sets Ebola and other viruses like it far apart from other diseases such as heart disease, hypertension, and cancer. Comparisons of fatalities due to EVD to those from other diseases are sometimes made to try to make the point that fears about EVD are "hyped." Such comparisons miss a critical factor: Ebola has much greater potential for rapid, progressive devastation than other disease. To think about this in terms of epidemiology, you have to take both geographic and demographic factors into account. In terms of its devastation, Ebola is like an earthquake that spreads. Even after the curve is bent, the risk of sporadic resurgence is very real. The death toll due to EVD includes deaths due to cases of other illnesses that go untreated because patients are afraid to go to the doctor for fear of being diagnosed with EVD, and for fear of contracting EVD. Deaths due to malaria in areas with EVD have soared. To see Ebola unleash itself on major cosmopolitan centers of the world such as Tokyo, Delhi, New York, Mexico City or Sao Paulo would be terrible; to see it take hold in any of the world's *densest* cities (for example: Dhaka, Hyerabad, Mumbai, Hong Kong) — now that would be terrifying.

The first EVD patient in US was Mr. Thomas Eric Duncan. Duncan contracted the disease in his home country Liberia, where he helped transport a woman sick with Ebola to a hospital. Duncan allegedly knew he had been exposed, and flew from Liberia to Brussels, then on to Washington, D.C., and then to Dallas, Texas. When he began to show symptoms of EVD, he arrived at the Texas Health Presbyterian Hospital complaining of headache, nausea and abdominal pain. He failed to tell the attending nurses and doctor that he had recently traveled from Liberia, and, according to information provided by employees involved, he was not asked. Two nurses attending became infected. CG Environmental, the company that cleaned up 140 drums of waste from Thomas Eric Duncan's apartment in Texas, estimated the cost of decontamination to be US$100,000. In the case study publication (Lowe *et al.*, 2014), the estimated volume of solid waste per patient was 50 pounds of solid waste per day (23 cubic feet). Most of this waste comprised of personal protective equipment (PPE) worn by attendant health care workers. Autoclaving was used to sterilize PPE, patient linens, scrubs, and towel and packaged for disposal as category B medical waste. Patients have been observed to produce on average 2.3 gallons of liquid waste per day, which was disposed of by being held in a toilet for 2.5 times the recommended time in disinfectant, before flushing the waste, exceeding CDC requirements. The WHO requirements for disposal are more lax, and this is a concern (Kibby *et al.*, 2014).

The cost for Duncan's care has been estimated at $500,000. This does include the settlement from the hospital to his family. The amount of resources that would be consumed to treat 34 million cases of Ebola would be unthinkably enormous. There are roughly one billion cases of viral hepatitis worldwide. Recall also that HIV and hepatitis are communicable over many years. Ebola is thought to be communicable during the symptomatic phase, up to, and after death, and for some time, averaging an infectious period of 2.58 days (Stadler *et al.*, 2014) but ranging as high as three weeks for the convalescent. For these reasons, few feel reassured by a low basic R0 for Ebola (see below).

Apparently neither does the CDC. In early December 2014, they announced that 35 hospitals in the US have been designated as Ebola Treatment Centers. They did not do this for HIV, or for hepatitis. They did this due to the concern that the number of infected patients in the US may eventually exceed the capacity of the existing four biocontainment clinical units. They also recently spent $27 million to secure personal protective equipment (PPEs).

Lest anyone suggest that this perspective is fear mongering, let us examine what this would mean in terms of other diseases with similar levels of communicability. Communicable diseases are rated on their ability to spread: This is called the basic reproductive rate (average number of transmissions per case during the communicable phase of the disease, assuming everyone in the population is susceptible). Ebola thus far has been rated at 1 to 4, at different stages of the epidemic; the range covers the likely number of people likely to be infected by a person with Ebola. Early estimates for R0 for the Sierra Leone outbreak vary between 1.7 (Gire *et al.*, 2014) and 2.2 (WHO Ebola Response Team, 2014). These numbers will vary with geography, with our responses, and will be refined as the epidemiological analysis continues.

Compare the R0 of EVD to that of polio (R0 5 to 7), diphtheria (6 to 7), measles (12 to 18), pertussis (12 to 17), mumps (4 to 7), HIV (1 to 4), and viral hepatitis (1 to 2), and we see where EVD stands in terms of the rate at which it is likely to spread. Comparisons to these numbers are often used to make the case that Ebola is not that dangerous; that representations of its manifestation and characterizations of Ebola that invoke fear are somehow irresponsible. That might be true if Ebola did not kill so efficiently, and in such as messy way. Let's assume Ebola has a R0 of somewhere between 1 and 4, depending on good, and bad, local conditions. That's a large range; even a small difference in R0 values can dramatically change projections. However, it is similar to that of HIV. In 2014, there were just over 34 million people living with HIV infections worldwide. Their care is now mostly pharmacological. Further, once a person is diagnosed as HIV-positive, they take care to reduce the risk of transmission to others via relatively simple behavioral changes. Thirty-four million Ebola-positive people in the world would not nearly as easily control the risk of transmission to others because they shed the virus in an uncontrolled manner. The patients are weak with lethargy, unable to walk, barely able to crawl as the virus decimates muscles, nerves, blood cells, and blood vessel walls. At much smaller numbers (thousands), care for new cases in some areas is palliative. The symptoms present suddenly, and there is little time — a matter of days — between the onset of first symptoms to a period of utter and total dependence on others for every basic need. Patient can unwittingly spread the virus all over the room when they are sick, and their bodies are highly contagious after death. This does not sound like HIV.

Scientists can still learn a lot from R0, from how many generations of transmission have probably taken place, to the likely size of the eventual outbreak. They can also study the projected effectiveness of measures to control an outbreak. Fisman *et al.* (2014) projected that three to four million doses of vaccine would be needed to be most effective for helping to control EVD in Western Africa by January/February 2015, but noted that vaccination might still be effective as late as July 2015. In Africa, cultures vary quite a bit, from isolated rural communities to very dense population centers in national capitals. The transmission rate is a function of interpersonal habits, hygiene practices, population density, and the intrinsic biology of the virus and its effects on the human body. Our ability to understand the relative importance of these factors is determined, in part, by the accuracy and completeness of the data. Under-reporting can influence estimates of R0. I spoke with Jeffrey Townsend, one of the authors of a study published in December 2014 of the R0 of Ebola under two assumptions: Random social association, and social clustering (Scarpino *et al.*, 2014). Dr. Townsend and his colleagues showed that, for the initially available data during the outbreak, under-reporting was perhaps not as severe as had been previously estimated. Their analysis also showed that previous R0 estimates may have been overestimated as the initial analyses did not sufficiently account for the social clustering evident in transmission chains.

The long-term differences in projections change dramatically with changes in R0. The value of R0 is influenced by a large number of factors. Generally, it differs with region, and whether there have been interventions or not. The value of R0 also differs when one analyses patients who survive separately from those who do not. The values early in the 2014 epidemic in Liberia were estimated to be 0.66 for survivors and 2.36 for non-survivors (Yamin *et al.*, 2014).

While I was discussing these numbers with Jeff in mid-December, he hastened to remind me that these figures are what analysts call "fit to data"; that is, they are based on certain assumptions, and on the accuracy and completeness of the data. The phylodynamic analyses that epidemiologists use during modern outbreaks are remarkable; events in the viral transmission chains are known from contact tracing; the mutations can be mapped, and the rate of spread, or decline of the rate of spread, is not subsumed into one number. Jeff would be the first to say that as much as goes into estimating R0, it is a guide, and really a snapshot in a dynamic process. For example, the same value of R0 at between two outbreaks can have different fates, depending on the momentum of events, as well.

Nevertheless, the measures are clearly useful for epidemiologists, public health officials, and health care workers: They provide an index that can guide response planning; projections are that the isolation of 75% of people within three to four days of the onset of symptoms, and safe burial of 75% of the dead, are key to stopping the epidemic. More recent modeling in Liberia may be cause for optimism in that country. Extensive modeling results from Drake *et al.* (2015) suggest that if isolation of 85% of the sick (via hospitalization) can be achieved in Liberia, the number of cases could be brought to zero (in Liberia only). The study, published in mid-January 2015, also found that both changes in individual behavior and increased success in hospitalization are key to bringing the numbers to zero. Other studies had previously listed many factors that play a role in stopping the epidemic, specifically "surveillance, case investigation, laboratory confirmation, contact tracing, safe transportation of persons with suspected Ebola, isolation, infection control within the health care system, community engagement, and safe burial" (Nyenswah *et al.*, 2014).

This is a leviathan effort. A diagnostic capable of detecting *Ebolavirus* in saliva prior to symptoms would be even better: It could allow treatment prior to symptoms, preventing symptoms and reducing the contagiousness. If the virus harbors early in the spleen, perhaps a biopsy test is worth the risk.

Some (like the US CDC) have taken the news that there may be fewer hidden cases than previously thought as an indication that we might not have to be as concerned as earlier expected. This is a dangerous interpretation. Even an R0 of 1.2 for a disease like EVD is an immense cause of concern. Combine the characteristics of exponential spread with the woeful state of non-preparedness for this epidemic in general, add the fact that resurgence is a clear possibility, and the result suggests that we might have a few months' time before we need to become as concerned as we thought might have to be. In the face of uncertainty on the effectiveness of the control measures that are being attempted, and the time it takes to ramp up support for control interventions, we should be as concerned now as we might have to be in a few months. If we are wrong in our preparations, and if the projections on containment prove optimistic, we should at least err in the correct direction.

There are many ways that transmission rates can be lowered; a list is provided at the end of this chapter. It is suspected that certain cultural practices, which vary greatly among different peoples in Western African countries, may have contributed initially in the outbreak to transmission rates much higher than 1 to 4. One oft-cited example is preparing the deceased for burial. An outbreak in Mali is thought to have been caused by the washing of the body of a deceased Guinean Imam, suspected of dying from the EVD on October 27 in Bamako, Mali, who had flu-like symptoms but who did not report visiting with or spending time with anyone known to have EVD or EVD-like symptoms. Another is a type of "wailing" during mourning, where the victim's family are in intimate contact with their loved one's body, embracing, washing the mouth, and clipping the finger nails. This is risky business when EVD is around, but it is still a procedure sacred to its participants. Some have emphasized that these practices should not be referred to in such a way as to sound alien, exotic, or foreign; all cultures prepare their loved ones for burial.

Taking care of those sick from Ebola is also very risky business. Those who do the most intimate care are more likely to become infected. This means that the virus is more likely to find female victims. Around 60% of all Ebola cases in the current outbreak are women (Wolfe, 2014). Casual contact has been downplayed by the CDC for EVD transmission in the US. Other cultural practices, which are less dramatic than burying the dead, also transmit the virus, such as shaking hands. People, including health care workers and public health personnel, now use an elbow bump to reduce person-to-person physical contact.

Dr. Gavin MacGregor-Skinner is a public health expert who works at the Department of Public Health Sciences at Penn State University, and is Global Projects Manager at the Elizabeth R. Griffin Research Foundation.. I learned from Gavin, during a phone interview, that to avoid infecting the mucous membranes of the eyes, nose, and mouth, newcomers in the field are advised to not raise their hands above their shoulders, which is a surprisingly difficult challenge.

The size of the outbreak in some countries in Western Africa makes government-imposed isolation difficult. The US CDC's guidance for self-monitoring of people potentially infected with *Ebolavirus* assumes that people are not contagious until they are symptomatic. It also assumes that infected people will follow the guidance. The data, to date, assures us that people will break their self-monitoring and professional and social distancing. In a study of an outbreak of norovirus in one hospital, one-third of the health care workers who were supposed to avoid other people to stop the spread of the disease did not do so (Rao *et al.*, 2009). Certainly experience in Africa, and in the US has shown that a percentage of people who are likely to be infected including health care workers, will not always act in a manner consistent with safe-guarding public health, and will violate their self-monitoring and isolation protocols.

During their time caring for EVD patients, health care workers treating EVD patients should be constantly monitored; ideally, there would be a near-instant exposure test. In a properly conducted care session, of donning and doffing of PPG, a buddy system is used, with a checklist, and if the procedures go off protocol, the partici-pants are made to stop so corrective action can take place. These processes, says Gavin, are absolutely critical to reducing the risk of infection to health care works. This is where drilling is so important. To isolate the risk of within-hospital transmissions, the US military is building Ebola wards in Western African countries to help isolate these treatment centers to reduce incidental exposure and spread.

EVD survivors should be constantly monitored as well. Given the findings of a WHO study that found outlying cases of infection occurring beyond 21 days, current expectations are that two successive negative tests after 42 days of contracting the disease means that a patient is Ebola-free. This recommendation is based on the study that showed that 98% of people infected with Ebola have an incubation period that falls within 42 days (WHO Ebola situation assessment, Oct 14, 2014). Patients can remain infectious after the incubation period, thus the common practice of 21 day isolation is in question. However, the 42-day mark is not without question. Three studies have found Ebola in the semen of convalescing men, for 40 days in samples from the outbreak in Gulu, Uganda in 2000 (Bausch *et al.*, 2007), 61 days in a case of laboratory infection in England (Edmond *et al.*, 1977), and 82 days in Kikwit, Democratic Republic of the Congo (Rodriguez *et al.* 1999). Although the Kikwit study reported no known instances of transmission from semen (Rowe *et al.*, 1999), as a result of these studies, the WHO recently advised that men cured of EVD abstain from sex, including oral sex, for a minimum of three months, but the risk may be longer. Data on the persistence of *Ebolavirus* in semen, vaginal secretions, and breast milk are scarce, but it is likely higher because these tissue compartments are immunologically protected sites with delayed viral clearance (Sonnenberg and Field, 2014). Research on transmission rates via these routes is needed. It is less known that current policy guidances of 42 days ignore the report from Kortepeter *et al.* (2011) that *Ebolavirus* can reside in the anterior chamber of the eye for weeks or even months after infection.

In 2012, quick-thinking medical teams at the Ministry of Health in Uganda starting tallying the clinical symptoms of patients suffering from possible Marburg virus and Ebola infections (Mbonye *et al.*, 2012). At the time, and until 2014, Marburg virus disease and Ebola hemorrhagic fever were, and by some still are, considered clinically indistinguishable. The team reported the following statistics: fever, 94.1%; headache, 70.6%; weakness, 64.7%; diarrhea, 47.1%; abdominal pain, 64.7%; vomiting, 14%, and bleeding, 35.1%. Data reported in a study in the *New England Journal of Medicine* from the 2014 outbreak (Schieffelin *et al.*, 2014) seems to show similar percentages of fever (89%), headache (80%), weakness (66%), and diarrhea (51%). However, in 2014, the percentages are lower for abdominal pain (40%) and bleeding elsewhere (<1%). Importantly, and not really reported anywhere to my knowledge, based on a comparison of these published data, the percentage of vomiting is much higher in the 2014 study (34%) than in the 2012 study (14%). In a more thorough analysis with more data (WHO Ebola Response Team, October 2014), vomiting in 2014 from Guinea, Liberia and Sierra Leone was up to 67.6%, abdominal pain was 44%, and bleeding was lower (hemorrhagic, <1% to 5.7%; unexplained bleeding, 18%). These symptoms may indicate a difference in the viral biology: The suspected increased risk of transmission may be related to these shifts.

Others are not quite ready to draw inferences from these data, and see the interpretation as speculative. During my discussions with him, Dr. Michael Osterholm, director of the Center for Infectious Disease Research and Policy at the University of Minnesota, told me that one has to be very careful in drawing conclusions from symptomological data from outbreaks of EVD given the haphazard manner in which the data are collected. He also cited high variability of symptoms within outbreaks, and across regions.

Human behavior, including that of patients and health care workers, is an important factor that influences transmission rates. It is important in two ways: First, it introduces opportunities for transmission, and second, we can modulate it to reduce risk. The viral phenotypes are another important aspect, and clinical symptoms are an important class of viral phenotypes, and human behavior — our reaction to the symptoms — is determined in part by the symptoms. Although EVD was initially called EHD, bleeding is not the only symptom that can spread the disease. If the symptomological data are indicative, then perhaps the combination of lower levels of abdominal pain associated with vomiting has increased the rate of spread by virtue of how caretakers are able to help the sick control the waste. Carefully conducted studies of the behavior of caretakers may help indicate points of transmission.

One way to die out if you're a virus is to be too virulent: A population of dead hosts is of no use to a virus. This virus tampers with and ultimately sabotages the human host's immune system long enough to gain a foothold in the host until it becomes unstoppably virulent. A recent study of HIV showed that it has become *less* easily

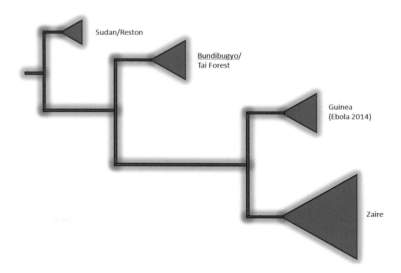

Fig. 1.2 Evolutionary story of the origins of Ebola guinea (*Guinea ebolavirus?*) as indicated by genomic sequence analysis (Baize *et al.*, 2014). Rooting of the tree was determined using outgroup analysis (with the placement of Sudan and Reston providing an indication of the "direction" of the tree). In this analysis, a robust clustering of the Guinea sequences, Ebola guinea, is evident and it seems separate from the *Zaire ebolavirus*. This placement does not require that Ebola guinea be viewed as derived from *Zaire ebolavirus* and is consistent with it being a distinct strain.

transmissible as we become more adept at diagnosis and treatment (Payne *et al.*, 2014). The change has been attributed to a loss of the ability of the HIV to overwhelm the immune system: It is becoming less virulent. It could also be due, in part, to the more widespread availability of antiretroviral drugs, but the Payne study saw a resistance to an HLA component of the human immune system. Whether this will continue to be the trend for HIV is unknown.

What about *Ebolavirus*? Is it showing other signs of changing phenotype? Gire *et al.* (2014) noted a large increase in the substitution rate of Ebola guinea compared to previous outbreaks. They also noted a protein-changing substitution in an RNA editing site of the glycoprotein (GP) gene. Dudas and Rambaut (2014) noted

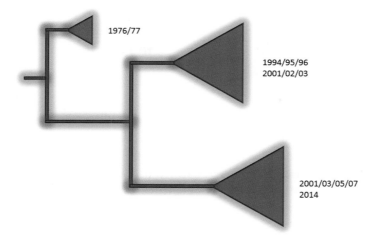

1976/77

1994/95/96
2001/02/03

2001/03/05/07
2014

Fig. 1.3   Rough outline of the evolutionary story of *Ebolavirus* since 1976, assuming time points to the root of the tree. This phylogenetic tree is derived from Dudas and Rambaut (2014), who rooted their phylogenetic estimations using a technique called "temporal rooting." In all published analyses, the Ebola guinea strains form a robust, distinct clade within the larger clade (not shown in this simplified representation).

two distinct clades when rooting the phylogenetic tree using time as the axis of the rooting of the tree. Is this the same as the old strain? Or is it a new strain, derived from the old with an accelerated mutation rate? Or, perhaps it is long-isolated from those behind past outbreaks? Their temporal rooting suggests it is recently derived; however the inference is potentially circular. With temporal rooting, the latest sequences would naturally fall on the directed graph as derived, so the rooting of the tree remains something of an open question. However, the robustness of the 2014 clade away from *Zaire ebolavirus* is found in all analyses. Within the 2014 clade, three main subgroups exist; recent genetic evidence suggests that the clade that made the border to Sierra Leone has traveled back to Guinea and Liberia and may have replaced the two other clades. Based on these analyses, and on the large phenotypic shifts in the disease symptomology, it appears safe

Table 1.2   Reducing Transmission of *Ebolavirus*. (Compiled from Various Sources.)

Do

Wash your hands frequently

Avoid large public gatherings

Avoid facilities where EVD patients are being treated, unless the facility is an ETU

Self-isolate if you suspect you have been exposed

Self-isolate if you develop fever, fatigue, headache, muscle pain, diarrhea, vomiting, stomach pain, or unexplained bruising or bleeding

At the first sign of symptoms, seek immediate medical care at an Ebola treatment center

Isolate your pets if they have been exposed

Do Not

Shake hands, or high-five

Touch body fluids from infected persons

Have sex with Ebola-infected persons

Handle items that may have come into contact with an infected person's blood or body fluids

If you are near an EVD patient, do not touch your face

Touch dead animals

Touch bats, or non-human primates

Forage, prepare, or consume animal carcasses from the forest

Transport the sick

Touch dead bodies

Eat raw meat prepared from bats or non-human primates

If treating EVD patients, bring your hands above your shoulders

Share dinner plates

Share blankets with people with flu-like symptoms

Donate blood to a blood bank if you think you have been exposed

to conclude that this virus is not *Zaire ebolavirus*. Until those responsible for viral systematics and nomenclature determine a name for it (such as *Guinea ebolavirus*), the three main clades of virus are, to me, Ebola guinea.

References

Adu-Gyamfi E, Soni SP, Jee CS, *et al.* (2014) A loop region in the N-terminal domain of Ebola virus VP40 is important in viral assembly, budding, and egress. *Viruses* **6(10):** 3837–54. doi: 10.3390/v6103837.

Althaus CL. (2014) Estimating the reproduction number of Ebola virus (EBOV) during the 2014 outbreak in West Africa. *PLOS Currents Outbreaks.* 2014 Sep 2. Edition 1. doi: 10.1371/currents.outbreaks.91 afb5e0f279e7f29e7056095255b288.

Audet J, Kobinger GP. (2014) Immune Evasion in Ebolavirus Infections. *Viral Immunol,* Nov 14, 2014.

Basler CF, Mikulasova A, Martinez-Sobrido L, *et al.* (2003) The Ebola virus VP35 protein inhibits activation of interferon regulatory factor 3. *J Virol* **77(14):** 7945–56.

Bausch D. *et al.* (2007) Assessment of the risk of Ebola virus transmission from bodily fluids and fomites. *J Infect Dis* **196:** S142–7.

Bornholdt ZA, *et al.* (2013) Structural rearrangement of Ebola virus VP40 begets multiple functions in the virus life cycle. *Cell* **154:** 763–74. doi: 10.1016/j.cell.2013.07.015.

Brauburger K, Boehmann Y, Tsuda Y, *et al.* (2014) Analysis of the highly diverse gene borders in Ebola virus reveals a distinct mechanism of transcriptional regulation. *J Virol* **88(21):** 12558–71. doi: 10.1128/JVI.01863-14.

Cárdenas WB, Loo YM, Gale M Jr, *et al.* (2006) Ebola virus VP35 protein binds double-stranded RNA and inhibits alpha/beta interferon production induced by RIG-I signaling. *J Virol* **80(11):** 5168–78.

Cook JD, Lee JE. (2013) The secret life of viral entry glycoproteins: Moonlighting in immune evasion. *PLOS Pathog* **9(5):** e1003258. doi: 10.1371/journal.ppat.1003258.

Drake JM, Kaul RB, Alexander LW, *et al.* (2015) Ebola cases and health system demand in Liberia. *PLOS Biol* **13(1):** e1002056. doi: 10.1371/journal.pbio.1002056.

Edmond, R. *et al.* (1977) A case of Ebola virus infection. *Br Med J* **2:** 541–44.

Fisman D, Khoo E, Tuite A. (2014) Early Epidemic Dynamics of the West African 2014 Ebola Outbreak: Estimates Derived with a Simple

Two-Parameter Model. *PLOS Currents: Outbreaks.* Sept 8, 2014. Edition 1. doi: 10.1371/currents.outbreaks.89c0d3783f36958d96eb bae97348d571.

Fisman D, Tuite A. (2014) Projected Impact of Vaccination Timing and Dose Availability on the Course of the 2014 West African Ebola Epidemic. *PLOS Currents Outbreaks.* Nov 21, 2014. Edition 1. doi: 10.1371/currents.outbreaks.06e00d0546ad426fed83ff24a1d4c4cc.

Gire SK, Goba A, Andersen KG, *et al.* (2014) Genomic surveillance elucidates Ebola virus origin and transmission during the 2014 outbreak. *Science* **345(6202):** 1369–72. doi: 10.1126/science.1259657.

Johnson SR. (2014) Clumsy Ebola response tests country's faith in health leaders. *Mod Healthc* **44(43):** 12. PubMed PMID: 25509614.

Lamb RA, Parks GD. (2007) Paramyxoviridae: the viruses and their replication. In: Knipe DM, Howley PM (eds), *Fields Virology*, Lippincott/ Williams & Wilkins, Philadelphia, pp. 1449–1498.

Leung LW, Hartman AL, Martinez O, *et al.* (2006) Ebola virus VP24 binds karyopherin α1 and blocks STAT1 nuclear accumulation. *J Virol* **80:** 5156–67.

Lowe J, Gibbs S, Schwedhelm S, *et al.* (2014) Nebraska Biocontainment Unit perspective on disposal of Ebola medical waste. *Am J Infect Cont* Vol 42, Dec 12, 2014.

Martínez MJ, Biedenkopf N, Volchkova V, *et al.* (2008) Role of Ebola virus VP30 in transcription re-initiation. *J Virol* **82(24):** 12569–73. doi: 10.1128/JVI.01395-08.

Mbonye A, Wamala J, Winyi-Kaboyo, *et al.* (2012) Repeated outbreaks of viral hemorrhagic fevers in Uganda. *Afr Health Sci* **12(4):** 579–83.

Mehedi M, Falzarano D, Seebach J, *et al.* (2011) A new Ebola virus nonstructural glycoprotein expressed through RNA editing. *J Virol* **85(11):** 5406–14. doi: 10.1128/JVI.02190-10.

Muhlberger E, Trommer S, Funke C, *et al.* (1996) Termini of all mRNA species of Marburg virus: sequence and secondary structure. *Virology* **223:** 376–80.

Noda T, Ebihara H, Muramoto Y, *et al.* (2006) Assembly and budding of Ebolavirus. *PLOS Pathog* **Sept; 2(9):** e99.

Nyenswah T, Fahnbulleh M, Massaquoi M, *et al.* (2014) Centers for Disease Control and Prevention (CDC). Ebola epidemic — Liberia,

March-October 2014. *Morb Mortal Wkly Rep* **63(46)**: 1082–6. Erratum in: *Morb Mortal Wkly Rep* **63(46)**: 1094.

Payne R, Muenchhoff M, Mann J, *et al.* (2014) Impact of HLA-driven HIV adaptation on virulence in populations of high HIV seroprevalence. *Proc Natl Acad Sci USA* **111(50)**: E5393-400. doi: 10.1073/pnas.1413339111.

Radzimanowski J, Effantin G, Weissenhorn W. (2014) Conformational plasticity of the Ebola virus matrix protein. *Protein Sci* **23(11)**: 1519–27. doi: 10.1002/pro.2541.

Rodriguez L. *et al.* (1999) Persistence and genetic stability of Ebola virus during the outbreak in Kikwit, Democratic Republic of Congo, 1995. *J Infect Dis* **179(1)**: S170–6.

Rowe A, *et al.* (1999) Clinical, virologic, and immunologic follow-up of convalescent Ebola hemorrhagic fever patients and their household contacts, Kikwit, Democratic Republic of the Congo. *J Infect Dis* **179(1)**: S28–35.

Scarpino SV, *et al.* (2014) Epidemiological and viral genomic sequence analysis of the 2014 Ebola outbreak reveals clustered transmission. *Clin Infect Dis.* doi: 10.1093/cid/ciu1131.

Schieffelin JS, *et al.* (2014) Clinical illness and outcomes in patients with Ebola in Sierra Leone. *N Engl J Med* **371(22)**: 2092–100. doi: 10.1056/NEJMoa1411680.

Sullivan, N, Yang Z-Y, Naebl GJ. (2003) Ebola virus pathogenesis: implications for vaccines and therapies. *J Virol* **77**: 9733–9737.

Volchkova VA, Klenk HD, Volchkov VE. (1999) Delta-peptide is the carboxy-terminal cleavage fragment of the nonstructural small glyco-protein sGP of Ebola virus. *Virology* **265**: 164–1.

Watanabe S, Noda T, Kawaoka Y. (2006) Functional mapping of the nucleoprotein of Ebola virus. *J Virol* **80**: 3743–51.

Wauquier N, Becquart P, Padilla C, *et al.* (2010) Human fatal zaire Ebola virus infection is associated with an aberrant innate immunity and with massive lymphocyte apoptosis. *PLOS Negl Trop Dis* **2010; 4**: e837. doi: 10.1371/journal.pntd.0000837.

WHO (2014) WHO Ebola situation assessment — Oct 14, 2014. [http://www.who.int/mediacentre/news/ebola/14-october-2014/en/]

WHO Ebola Response Team. (2014) Ebola virus disease in West Africa — the first 9 months of the epidemic and forward projections. *N Engl J Med.* [http://dx.doi.org/10.1056/NEJMoa1411100]

Yamin D, Gertler S, Ndeffo-Mbah ML, *et al.* (2014) Effect of Ebola progression on transmission and control in Liberia. *Ann Int Med* **162(1):** 11–7. doi: 10.7326/M14-2255.

Zhang AP, Bornholdt ZA, Liu T, *et al.* (2012) The Ebola virus interferon antagonist VP24 directly binds STAT1 and has a novel, pyramidal fold. *PLOS Pathog* e1002550. doi: 10.1371/journal.ppat.1002550.

2

How Well Do We Understand the 2014 *Ebolavirus*?

> *There's zero doubt in my mind that barring a mutation which changes it — which we don't think is likely — there will not be a large outbreak in the US. We know how to control Ebola, even in this period. I would be very concerned if there were mutations in this virus. There are none.*

That was the Q&A testimony provided to the US House Oversight Hearings on Ebola in October by Dr. Thomas Frieden, Director of the CDC.

Much of the political discussion of "mutation" to date in the Ebola crisis appears to have focused on the possibility that this strain *will* mutate. These questions are usually addressed by a referral back to the priority of dealing with the containment of Ebola in Western Africa.

But another question may prove to be even more pressing: What if this strain has already mutated?

Scientists looking at the sequences see differences between the 2014 strain and past sequences of *Zaire ebolavirus*. Mutations. Plenty of them.

> *Because many of the mutations alter protein sequences and other biologically meaningful targets, they should be monitored for impact on diagnostics, vaccines, and therapies critical to outbreak response.* (Gire *et al.*, 2014).

We find evidence for adaptive evolution affecting L and GP protein coding regions of the EBOV genome. (Volz and Pond, 2014).

This study demonstrates the emergence of a new EBOV strain in Guinea. (Baize *et al.*, 2014.)

Here we find evidence that major Sierra Leone clades have systematic differences in growth rate and reproduction number. (Luska *et al.*, 2014).

Medicine and science are both imperfect arts. There are significant gaps in our biological knowledge in most areas of medicine. And yet we in the public rely heavily upon medical experts for our diagnoses and treatments. In the last decade, I have seen the emergence of knowledge that should be applied to change medical practice, but the practice goes on unaltered. This occurs for various reasons, but to researchers, it's called failed translation; to economists, it's called market failure. Many times only those treatments that can lead to profit make it to market. To some, this is a matter-of-fact business. The practice of failure-to-translate is, in my opinion, the scourge of modern western medicine. Two examples come to mind, both related to breast cancer, and both very personal. My sister was diagnosed with breast cancer in November 2008. We have a serious problem of both incidence and penetrance of breast cancer among women on the maternal side of my family; my mom died in 1971 at the age of 33; her sister was diagnosed and survived after a bilateral radical mastectomy. My aunt's daughters, unfortunately, both passed from breast cancer at the age of 25. Poverty played a role in the neglect of their cancer, but it had help. My family has a BRCA1 variant segregating that, while not yet recognized as a clinical mutation, results in nine amino acids being missing from the BRCA1 protein. It's a nine amino acid deletion, so I am fairly sure it has a large influence on the protein's function. My sister's cancer was triple negative (ER, PR, and Her-2 Neu), which tends to be aggressive, and hard to treat: It does not express the hormone receptors that many available chemotherapy agents target.

The first example of existing knowledge ignored by the medical community involves the so-called breast cancer genes, BRCA1 and BRCA2, and the risk of cancer from mammography. BRCA1 is a DNA repair enzyme that works to repair double-stranded breaks in DNA — the type induced by X-rays. A study in 1996 (Goldfrank *et al.*, 1996) showed a higher incidence of breast cancer in women who had BRCA1 or BRCA2 mutations and underwent mammography. This study alone should have caused breast cancer specialists everywhere to encourage patients with familial breast cancer to get tested for BRCA1 and BRCA2 mutations, and to stay away from mammography if the women in their family with breast cancer have a BRCA1 or BRCA2 mutation. I mentioned this issue in an editorial I published in 2008, but have never seen any formal study of this obvious risk factor for some women. However, GINA (the Genetic Information Nondiscriminatory Act) was not passed until 2008, so between 1996 and 2008, the translational opportunity was lost. During this time, I had insisted that my sister get mammograms.

The second example is the continued use of low-dose tamoxifen as a long-term prophylactic to protect against recurrent breast cancer. Tamoxifen targets the estrogen receptor (ER). My sister's cancer, being triple negative, expressed no ER. She asked me to call her oncologist, as I had questioned the wisdom of this prescription. I asked him politely to describe the need of a low-dose tamoxifen prescription for my sister. To protect against the recurrence of breast cancer, he said. I then asked him if he knew of any published study that had shown any protective benefit of low-dose tamoxifen on ER-negative breast cancer. The good doctor became very angry with me, admonished me to "go back to being my sister's brother, and stop trying to be her doctor," and hung up. When I relayed this reaction to a simple question to my sister, she decided to forego the treatment, and now, six years later, she has added two beautiful boys to her family. I don't know if that oncologist is still prescribing low-dose tamoxifen to women whose breast cancer was ER-negative, but I hope he is not.

The dismissive attitude of the oncologist occurred at a time when a parallel experience was occurring in my research life. I had made a discovery using a new machine learning technique called "Efficiency Analysis" (Jordan *et al.*, 2008). In this empirical technique for comparing methods of data analysis, high-dimensional genomic and proteomic data are subsampled repeatedly to determine the internal consistency or reproducibility of the selection of genes or proteins in terms of differential expression. I had discovered, quite by accident, that using ratio of expression values (tumor/normal) is biased: Large portions of the measurements are "invisible" to the analysis when a ratio was used, but they could be "seen" when a true measure of difference (e.g., tumor/normal) was used. I was uncertain of the validity of the results, and so I invited a select group of experts to the meeting. Most were impressed that efficiency analysis was so good at finding differences among methods for the analysis of microarray and other data.

A few understood that the result also showed a bias in fold-change. After the meeting, a friend came up to me; his sister had recently died from breast cancer. He told me that I could expect this finding to be very, very hard to accept by the community due to their past use of fold-change. He also told me that I was too optimistic about the utility of the type of methodological research I am fond of conducting:

> *Your problem, Jim, is that you think you can make a difference in cancer. I've been at this for 25 years, and the results don't matter. Grant funding matters. But the actual results are unlikely to change clinical practice.*

My heart was broken.

For all of his training and experience, my sister's oncologist had somehow missed the published literature that I had familiarized myself with due, in part, to my sister's cancer. And, importantly, he refused to be objective in the face of new information, which, for all I knew, must have seemed to him to come from left field. There are many, many examples in which cutting edge medical knowledge, well, needed updating, and where reliance on the known can cause patients to suffer and die. I once had a close oncologist friend tell me: "You know we kill patients with chemo all of the time, Jim. Sometimes it's a contest between the tumor and the patient to see who dies first." His frankness may shock some; it did me. But he is a passionate oncologist who fights every day for people's lives, constantly seeking improvements in their care and outcomes, and he, and his patients, must accept the risks of dose-related mortality and morbidity every day.

For reasons like this, medical doctors are expected to keep up with findings relevant to the treatment needs of their patients. For a particular condition like breast cancer, some doctors missing some of the nuances of managing chemo for the rarer subtypes of cancer might be understood by some. For me, and my sister, that doctor's blithe position with respect to such patients' exposure to a lifetime of unnecessary treatment was inexcusable. He knew the hormonal status of my sister's triple negative breast cancer, and yet he wanted to treat her, to protect against recurrence, with a drug that was known to not even target this type of cancer. Uterine and ovarian cancer are risks for my sister; tamoxifen may be a small risk factor for uterine cancer, and it is used to treat ovarian cancer. However, the question to the oncologist was in terms of recurrent breast cancer. He apparently did not have a sufficient grasp of the biology of hormone-receptor mediated chemotherapy options, was not sufficiently objective to reassess his decisions about his care of my sister, and women like her, when presented with presented with evidence that he was treating someone unnecessarily.

The question for all of us, at this time, is whether we truly have a sufficient grasp on the biology of this strain of Ebola compared to past outbreaks to determine, as was reported, that "we know this virus," and if the answer is "no," then are we objective enough to move forward?

The Ebola virus itself was first discovered in 1976; however, experts agree that it is almost certain not to be a new virus. Historical anecdotes exist in Eastern Africa of a terrible fever that caused trepidation among travelers from western countries.

Historical white explorers and naturalists in Africa often reported instances of mysterious diseases simply referred to as "fever." The perspective at the time was that Africa was raging with epidemics of mysterious illnesses that had no name but could kill quickly. Typhus was known as "putrid fever." US president Theodore Roosevelt had reservations about bringing his son Kermit on an expedition to Africa: "I have been a little worried about him in connection with the fever," he wrote (Jeffers, 2014). Roosevelt consulted with experts who advised him that areas other than East Africa might be safer, such as Uganda and the Upper Nile, where "the fever was not as bad." A variety of symptoms are consistent with multiple diseases. Vomiting black blood, for example, could have, at the time, have been routinely attributed to ulcers or yellow fever. Looking back at case histories of deaths reported from regions known to currently harbor Ebola in the wild, and the symptoms, and I think it is fair to speculate that many cases were misdiagnosed, as many still are today, as malaria or other diseases.

Our best understanding of the origins of the species *Zaire ebolavirus* strain is that it appears to have a very recent origin. An analysis of the substitution rates based on nucleotide differences among 97 genome sequences suggests that the species *Zaire ebolavirus* and *Reston ebolavirus* share a common ancestor, perhaps as recently as 50 years ago (Carroll *et al.*, 2013). Ebola guinea seems very different.

Let's take a look at some modern eyewitness accounts.

Dr. Michael Osterholm, in his presentation at Johns Hopkins University (Osterholm, 2014), cited reported incidences in 2014 in which patients progressed from infection to death without ever presenting with fever. He did not report this as typical, but it raises the question of whether we understand the virus. He also cited that considering all past outbreaks of *Ebolavirus*:

> *We've had roughly 2,400 cases of illness; that's in 40 years... this virus has hardly pinged the human species until now and yet we have this sense that we know so much about it... and maybe we do; but* **something has changed**.

In July 2014, when the number of cases numbered only in the hundreds, Liberia's Information Minister Lewis Brown said:

We do need all of the help we can get. We need hands, we need expertise, we need equipment, and yes we need money. We need counseling. Some of our health care workers are frightened. You can understand that not only is this unprecedented, we simply never had this kind of attack on our way of life before. (PRI, July 2014).

Referring to the production of the *Frontline* documentary "Ebola Outbreak," producer Wael Dabbous said in a press release (October, note emphasis added):

*We spent more than two weeks on the ground in Sierra Leone, and we were stunned by what we saw. This time — **unlike in past Ebola outbreaks** — the virus has spread so rapidly, to so many people, that traditional modes of containment can't keep up. Local hospitals are overwhelmed and barely functioning because so many doctors and nurses have died.* (Sefton, 2014; PBS *Frontline*, 2014).

Current estimates of the percentage of EVD deaths in health care workers are around 5% (WHO). In Sierra Leone, it's a whopping 7.5% (November 2014). Early on, the rate of health care worker infection seemed too high; it indicated to some, including me, that something was very different. By December 2014, 13 doctors had contracted the disease; of these, 11 had died. The situation was, and is, so bad that health care workers stay home. Health care workers have gone on strike, seeking safety improvements in an untenable situation. By all accounts, they are exhausted, and scared. The CDC is using copies of the *Frontline* documentary as part of the training of health care workers from the US and elsewhere as they travel to help care for the sick. A video game has been developed to train new health care workers in the donning and doffing of PPE.

The design of hospitals may be a contributing factor. Dr. Gavin MacGregor-Skinner told me that Ebola Treatment Units have to follow a strict design, or people will get sick. Your movements should be highly controlled. At the beginning of the work day, you enter a clean room; at the end of the day, you leave a hot room, and disinfect thoroughly. He said one hospital, built by a charity for exclusive use as an Ebola Treatment Unit, was closed down by the Red Cross as unsafe for use for the treatment of EVD.

Harvard research scientist Lisa Hensley and her colleagues, working in Liberia, found that Ebola particles in a much higher concentration in blood samples from patients in the 2014 compared to samples analyzed during previous outbreaks — another clue that this is not the Zaire strain (*The New Yorker*, Oct 27, 2014, "The Ebola Wars: How genomics research can help contain the outbreak").

Whatever the molecular and biological differences are, the observations and data all point to one key truth: This virus spreads faster than viruses from past outbreaks. Also, contrary to certain reports, the genomes of patients in this outbreak show distinct mutations compared to past outbreaks. Are these two differences related? There are numerous ways in which a virus can become more easily spread. Anything the virus can do to make the host shed more virions uncontrollably is likely the phenotype (biological characteristic) that causes high transmission frequencies. This include becoming more easily aerosolized (Piercy *et al.*, 2010). We know that droplet exposure in animals causes lethal infections (Formenty *et al.*, 2006; Jaax *et al.*, 1996). We also know that studies of aerosolized *Ebolavirus* have shown high transmissibility among animals via this route (Twenhafel *et al.*, 2014; Zumbrun *et al.*, 2012). Near airborne-like frequencies of transmission have been seen in pigs (Kobinger *et al.*, 2011). We will revisit the issue of transmission biology in more depth in the next chapter.

One of the characteristics of a virus that determines how many copies are made over time is the replication rate: The amount of time it takes to make one new copy of the virus. Replication rates depend on physical characteristics such as gene length, and protein size. For a given protein, for example, for most life forms, it also depends on transcription rates, which is how long it takes the cell to produce a copy of RNA that encode a protein. The rate of transcription also depends on the complexity of the local encoding DNA sequence. Perhaps some of these mutations cause faster rates of transcription by providing sufficient local complexity (mixes of nucleotides) and high disorder that the transcriptase zips along the RNAs at a faster rate. Alternatively, perhaps some of the mutations prevent the "normal" stuttering during transcription that leads to the sGP epitopes, causing the virus to abandon the strategy of providing distraction camouflage in favor of a faster replication rate, causing the virions to outnumber antibodies faster. Further, perhaps this small epitope not normally incorporated into the virus might be present, or perhaps there is an epitope missing.

Also, let's go back to the first patients. In the first few patients, we saw reports of bleeding in one patient, Emile's mother, Sia. After that, few instances of bleeding have been reported. Recall that the published data show that vomiting is much higher in 2014 (34%) than in 2012 (14%), and that fewer people bleed out. The *NEJM* study of the emergence, for which five of the co-authors on the study died from EVD, suggested the use of the term "Ebola virus disease" (EVD) as opposed to "Ebola hemorrhagic fever" to help clinicians and public health workers recognize the disease. It is tempting to speculate about a "molecular patient zero," either Emile, his sister, or his grandmother, in whom a new strain evolved that does not involve as much hemorrhaging.

If such a transition took place, it likely was not a new mutation, *per se*, but rather a shift in the quasispecies population frequencies of a specific genetic variant from low, to higher. But are these symptomological differences even real? An earlier study (Kortepeter *et al.*, 2011) summarizing symptoms from 1967–2013 for Marburg and Ebola reported that the majority of cases with bleeding were from the intestinal tract. Better data collection is needed for outbreaks to compare not just the genes, but the symptoms of diseases so the medical community can learn updated expectations for patients' needs.

The genetic differences in Ebola guinea cannot be dismissed out of hand for a lack of evidence that they have not changed the viral biology. It is an open question, and the possibility of a causal relationship between any potential differences in symptoms deserves closer, full, and exhaustive scientific scrutiny. Viruses shed in the mucous of a patient can be spread by sneezing, coughing and other means. Another smart way for this Ebola could spread farther, and faster would be to not causing the victim to bleed out and die, displaying a sure sign of infectivity, but instead to undergo long bouts of illness shedding virions in other ways that already exist — extended periods of vomiting, without the forewarning of abdominal pain, and diarrhea, for example. Perhaps we already have evidence of one or more culprits in the symptomology? Is this strain of the virus somehow better able to induce emissis? And, if it is real, how does the apparent increased incidence of vomiting effect transmission? We cannot dismiss this hypothesis due to a lack of data, rather, research should be conducted on the virus' ability to subterfuge the warning signs of vomiting, and its ability to spread more via its effects on the gastrointestinal tract.

Does the lower pH of the stomach acid aid in the transmission? *"We wash our PPGs and dry them in the sunlight to sterilize them, and re-use them,"* Dr. Gavin MacGregor-Skinner told me. What effect, if any, does stomach acid have on the PPGs, on transmissibility of the virus via skin? What about human behavior? Are people less averse to exposing themselves to vomitus from loved ones, than to blood? The questions add up: More detailed research on the disease phenotypes of EVD is needed.

Phylogenies Are Not Data

We know species by their characteristics, and by their genes. *Zaire ebolavirus,* of which the 2014 appears to be a very close relative, is the most deadly of these (mortality rates Zaire, 79%; *Sudan ebolavirus,* 53%; *Bundibugyo ebolavirus,* 27%; *Reston ebolavirus,* 0%; and *Tai forest ebolavirus* (originally *Côte d'Ivoire ebolavirus*), 0%; CDC data). The relationship of *Zaire* to other *Ebolavirus* discovered thus far was studied in 1997 by Georges-Courbot *et al.* (1997). Their tree was based on the sequences of the protein-encoding gene GP.

It shows large differences between different species, and very low (nearly no) variation within strains.

There are a few extremely important publications on the evolutionary and epidemiological analysis of Ebola guinea. They find the 2014 strain to be different, with surprisingly large amounts of variation among isolates from within the epidemic. Here are some quotes taken directly from the publications. I realize this is poor authorship, however, the time is pressing, and I hope to share as much as possible with each reader. I encourage all to read these papers in their entirety. Together, they report and underscore the message that perhaps we do not yet know the virus we're dealing with (emphasis via underlining and emboldening, mine):

> *In March 2014, the World Health Organization was notified of an outbreak of a communicable disease characterized by fever, severe diarrhea, vomiting, and a high fatality rate in Guinea. Virologic investigation identified Zaire ebolavirus (EBOV) as the causative agent. Full-length genome sequencing and phylogenetic analysis showed that EBOV from Guinea **forms a separate clade in relationship to the known EBOV strains from the Democratic Republic of Congo and Gabon.** Epidemiological investigation linked the laboratory-confirmed cases with the presumed first fatality of the outbreak in December 2013. **This study demonstrates the emergence of a new EBOV strain in Guinea.***
>
> — Baize *et al.* (2014) Emergence of Zaire Ebola Virus
> Disease in Guinea. *N Engl J Med* **371**: 1418–1425.
> doi: 10.1056/NEJMoa1404505.

> *Members of the genus Ebolavirus have caused outbreaks of hemorrhagic fever in humans in Africa. The most recent outbreak in Guinea, which began in February of 2014, is still ongoing. Recently published analyses of sequences from this outbreak suggest that the outbreak in Guinea is **caused by a divergent lineage of Zaire ebolavirus.** We report evidence that points to the same Zaire ebolavirus lineage that has previously caused outbreaks in the Democratic*

Republic of Congo, the Republic of Congo and Gabon as the culprit behind the outbreak in Guinea.

— Dudas G, Rambaut A. (2014) Phylogenetic Analysis of Guinea 2014 EBOV Ebolavirus Outbreak. *PLOS Currents: Outbreaks*, May 2, 2014.

doi:10.1371/currents.outbreaks.84eefe5ce43ec9dc0bf0670f7b8b417d.

*In its largest outbreak, Ebola virus disease is spreading through Guinea, Liberia, Sierra Leone, and Nigeria. We sequenced 99 Ebola virus genomes from 78 patients in Sierra Leone to ~2000× coverage. We observed a rapid accumulation of interhost and intrahost genetic variation, allowing us to characterize patterns of viral transmission over the initial weeks of the epidemic. This West African variant likely diverged from central African lineages around 2004, crossed from Guinea to Sierra Leone in May 2014, and has exhibited sustained human-to-human transmission subsequently, with no evidence of additional zoonotic sources. **Because many of the mutations alter protein sequences and other biologically meaningful targets, they should be monitored for impact on diagnostics, vaccines, and therapies critical to outbreak response.***

— Gire *et al.* (2014) Genomic surveillance elucidates Ebola virus origin and transmission during the 2014 outbreak. *Science* **345**: 1369–1372.

Background and Methodology: The current Ebola virus epidemic in West Africa has been spreading at least since December 2013. The first confirmed case of Ebola virus in Sierra Leone was identified on May 25. Based on viral genetic sequencing data from 72 individuals in Sierra Leone collected between the end of May and mid June, we utilize a range of phylodynamic methods to estimate the basic reproductive number (R0). We additionally estimate the expected lengths of the incubation and infectious periods of the virus. Finally, we use phylogenetic trees to examine the role played by population structure in the epidemic. Results: The median estimates of R0 based on sequencing data alone range between 1.65–2.18, with the most plausible model yielding a median R0 of 2.18 (95% HPD 1.24–3.55). Importantly, our results indicate that, at least until mid June, relief efforts in Sierra Leone were ineffective at lowering the effective reproductive number of the virus. We estimate the expected length of the infectious period to be 2.58 days (median; 95% HPD 1.24–6.98). The data set appears to be too small in order to estimate the incubation period with high certainty (median expected incubation period 4.92 days; 95% HPD 2.11–23.20). While our estimates of the duration of infection tend to be smaller than previously reported, phylodynamic analyses support a previous estimate that 70% of cases were observed and included in the present dataset. The dataset is too small to show a particular population structure with high significance, however our preliminary analyses suggest that half the population is spreading the virus with an R0 well above 2, while the other half of the population is spreading with an R0 below 1. Conclusions: Overall we show that sequencing data can robustly infer key epidemiological parameters. Such estimates inform public health officials and help to coordinate effective public health efforts. Thus having more sequencing data available for the ongoing Ebola virus epidemic and at the start of new outbreaks will foster a quick understanding of the dynamics of the pathogen.

— Stadler T, Kühnert D, Rasmussen DA, du Plessis L. (2014) Insights into the Early Epidemic Spread of Ebola in Sierra Leone Provided by Viral Sequence Data. *PLOS Currents: Outbreaks.*

doi:10.1371/currents.outbreaks.02bc6d927ecee7bbd33532ec8b a6a25f.*1*

Background: The Ebola virus (EBOV) epidemic in Western Africa is the largest in recorded history and control efforts have so far failed to stem the rapid growth in the number of infections. Mathematical models serve a key role in estimating epidemic growth rates and the reproduction number (R0) from surveillance data and, recently, molecular sequence data. Phylodynamic analysis of existing EBOV time-stamped sequence data may provide independent estimates of the unobserved number of infections, reveal recent epidemiological history, and provide insight into selective pressures acting upon viral genes. Methods: We fit a series mathematical models of infectious disease dynamics to phylogenies estimated from 78 whole EBOV genomes collected from distinct patients in May and June of 2014 in Sierra Leone, and perform evolutionary analysis on these genomes combined with closely related EBOV genomes from previous outbreaks. Two analyses are conducted with values of the latent period that have been used in recent modeling efforts. We also examined the EBOV sequences for evidence of possible episodic adaptive molecular evolution during the 2014 outbreak. Results: We find evidence for adaptive evolution affecting L and GP protein coding regions of the EBOV genome, which is unlikely to bias molecular clock and phylodynamic analyses. We estimate R0=2.40 (95% HPD:1.54–3.87) if the mean latent period is 5.3 days, and R0=3.81, (95% HPD:2.47–6.3) if the mean latent period is 12.7 days. The estimated coefficient of variation (CV) of the number of transmissions per infected host is very high, and a large proportion of infections yield no transmissions.

Conclusions: Estimates of R0 are sensitive to the unknown latent infectious period which cannot be reliably estimated from genetic data alone. EBOV phylogenies show significant evidence for superspreading and extreme variance in the number of transmissions per infected individual during the early epidemic in Sierra Leone.

— Volz E, Pond S. (2014) Phylodynamic Analysis of
Ebola Virus in the 2014 Sierra Leone Epidemic.
PLOS Currents: Outbreaks.

doi:10.1371/currents.outbreaks.6f7025f1271821d4c815385b08
f5f80e.1

The 2014 epidemic of the Ebola virus is governed by a genetically diverse viral population. In the early Sierra Leone outbreak, a recent study has identified new mutations that generate genetically distinct sequence clades. **Here we find evidence that major Sierra Leone clades have systematic differences in growth rate and reproduction number.** *If this growth heterogeneity remains stable, it will generate major shifts in clade frequencies and influence the overall epidemic dynamics on time scales within the current outbreak. Our method is based on simple summary statistics of clade growth, which can be inferred from genealogical trees with an underlying clade-specific birth–death model of the infection dynamics. This method can be used to perform realtime tracking of an evolving epidemic and identify emerging clades of epidemiological or evolutionary significance.*

— Łuksza M, Bedford T, Lässig M. (2014) Epidemiological and evolutionary analysis of the 2014 Ebola virus outbreak. arXiv:1411.1722 (submitted on Nov 6, 2014)

The total number of nucleotide variants cataloged in the *NEJM* study in initial patients from the outbreak was 396, 50 of which have the potential to alter the amino acid sequence, and thus the protein structure, and thus its function. The overall number of 396 and the placement of the 2014 clade in the tree as a derivative of the Zaire strain imply a mutation rate that appears to be twice that from between previous outbreaks. These differences are sufficient to cause Ebola guinea strains to cluster into a group of their own, distinct and separate from sequences from past outbreaks. Rooting a phylogenetic tree with accuracy can be challenging; nevertheless the published results and the analyses seem to indicate that the virus in West Africa is related to the Zaire strain, but is either *new*, or is at least distinct from, the Zaire strain. If the phylogenetic tree is correct in this respect, then we should be actively seeking a mechanistic explanation of an increased mutation rate of this strain compared to others, and concerned about where evolution might take this virus.

These analyses are exquisite, hard-won results (Fig. 2.1); the phylodynamic analysis (Łuksza *et al.*, 2014) especially adds a valuable dimension of genetic relatedness to the story of the transmission chain. It reveals the details of the trace analysis considering geography, genetics, and time — the initial spread within the 2014 is perhaps the best well-documented in history. It shows cleanly the increase in the mutation rate in the newest sequences. The timing of the transmission of Ebola guinea to humans is in little doubt, and within the outbreak, specific transmission events can be seen in the phylogenetic tree. So fine-grained is the analysis that individual events such as marriages and funerals can be pinpointed. A suspected dual infection was even observed; either two different quasispecies were transferred to one woman, or she was infected by two people.

Phylogenetic trees, however, are not observations; they are not "data," they are "results." When I was a graduate student, the field was more optimistic: Many, especially in the "parsimony" camp of phylogenetic methodology, like to refer to the process of phylogenetic inference as "reconstruction."

I have always preferred to think of the process as "estimation," for that's really what it is. The tree is a model of what might have happened, including branching order, and the amount of evolutionary

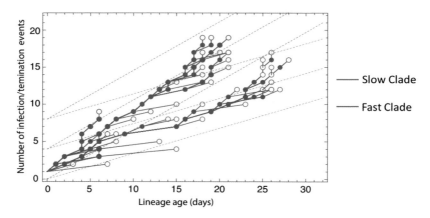

Fig. 2.1 Phylodynamic analysis of genomic sequences from Sierra Leone patients (Łuzska *et al.*, 2014). This analysis shows simultaneously the transmission chains and increase in the number of transmission events (x-axis) in the most recently derived isolates (red lines) compared to earlier isolates over the same analogous time period of disease spread (y-axis). Figure ©2014 Łuksza *et al.* Used with permission.

change is estimated between nodes. Uncertainty exists in every phylogenetic inference made using natural data, and my own research has shown that the estimates of branch lengths are not independent. In other words, every published tree is, arguably, incorrect in some details. This is widely known by researchers in phylogenetics and molecular systematics, and those in molecular evolution. For the most part, they hope that the trees are not incorrect in important details. Trees are inferred measures, and their accuracy is constrained by well-known factors. Each sequence, representing an isolate of Ebola, for example, must place somewhere in the tree, regardless of the overall tree's accuracy. This is not to draw into question whether the tree published in *NEJM* is correct overall. The phylogenetic clustering of all of the Ebola guinea sequences apart from *Zaire* has been shown to be robust, and is consistent with a single host-to-human transmission. The placement of that cluster, or clade, relative to the inferred "root" of the tree, however, is of extreme importance for the clinical and epidemiological implications of Ebola guinea. If the mutation rate of this strain has jumped dramatically, it means that the mutational process, which limits the rate of molecular evolution, will lead to increased numbers of variations in the population of *Ebolavirus* infecting people. Which direction the virus could travel in the future, both on the evolutionary and geographic landscapes, is unknown.

However, if the placement of the clade is due to one of a number of well-known artifacts in phylogenetic inference, a third explanation is possible. While the clustering suggests that the current strain is derived from the same wild reservoir as those from a past outbreak, it is possible that the virus is a long-isolated strain, related to Zaire strain, but not yet seen in humans. An error in the tree could mean a longer period of time for mutations to collect, and thus a slower rate of molecular evolution or one on par with that seen in past outbreaks. This less dire interpretation, however, is made less likely given that a team of researchers has seen evidence of the hammerhead bat migrating, dispersing the *Ebolavirus*. This is the same species of bat in Zaire. This bat species, as well as others, is well-suspected of being one of the most likely natural reservoirs of *Ebolavirus* (Quammen, 2014). Mark and recapture studies, albeit dangerous work, seem wise to track the migration patterns of these most likely reservoir species.

Regardless of the placement of the cluster or its age, the evolutionary distance — while <10%, the unofficial cut-off for calling a strain of Ebola a new "species" — is still larger than that seen between other outbreaks of the same strain. Because of the mutations that have been seen, my colleagues and I have taken to referencing to the 2014 strain as "Ebola zaire+," or "Ebola guinea," and hence the title of this book. The actual combined effects of the amino acid substitutions in various proteins on the viral biology of the *Ebolavirus* are as yet unknown, but they, too, must be studied as thoroughly and as soon as possible. The constant spread of the disease also makes new mutations more likely; these must be cataloged rapidly, and the massive amount of data interpreted in a systematic manner alongside the phenotypic data in search of any new mutations that may make Ebola guinea even more dangerous. The initial studies reveal some 300-odd mutations, with a total of 18 that change amino acids in the protein-coding sequences. Amino acid differences in one of the genes, Gp1Gp2, could in principle influence the immune system's ability to mount an antibody defense against the virus. Such variants, however, could prove useful for those developing diagnostic assays specific for Ebola guinea strains: Antibody-like molecules could be evolved that detect Ebola in general, accompanied by secondary molecules tuned to detect specific strains of Ebola. Given the large symptomological differences that can occur between strains, and the potential utility of this additional detail for contact tracing and for rapid molecular epidemiology, this approach would seem most prudent.

While sequencing is important, it is not enough to tally mutations. In this case, their functional significance must be studied and their effects on the viral phenotype understood. Association studies of specific variants with clinical outcomes, and with symptoms, would be an important place to start. Careful, detailed records of each patient's clinical course, the ordering and severity of symptoms, and their outcomes could be tallied in one massive international

EVD outcomes database, with identifiers matching clinical samples and sequence data derived from each patient.

Dealing with the lack of such a centralized database for clinical and epidemiological reporting and record-keeping is an important priority. Dr. Gavin MacGregor-Skinner decries how difficult it is to get reliable information about patients: Their symptoms, how they were treated, and their outcomes. Capturing this type of information is essential. Again, this is where he finds that western medical institutions appear to have fallen short of their potential.

> *We did not send the whole Ebola response team,* Gavin told me in our telephone interview. *We sent health care workers, but we did not send database specialists, IT support, and, importantly, data entry people. For us, we treat people all day, and then go to the hotel and enter data at night. A team dispatched to set up wireless networks, establish data entry routines is needed, otherwise we won't be able to make sense out of the processes in place and find out what worked best.*

Evolution Caught Red-handed

From a population genetics point of view, evolution, or more specifically, microevolution, is the gradual change in allele frequencies in a population over time. Alleles are specific nucleotides at specific base locations in an organism's genome. Viruses such as *Ebolavirus* and influenza exist as quasispecies: Even within a single patient, many variant strains can exist, either due to multiple infections, or, as is more commonly thought, evolutionary changes in copies of the virus carry new lineages away from the founding strain. If the immune system "sees" the viral strains, immunoselection, or antigenic pressure, can drive the changes in the frequencies of the strain from low numbers to becoming the predominant strain in a person, importantly, with a causal effect being the significance of the allele(s) driven to fixation to the survival and reproduction of the virus.

Evolution can also occur via random fluctuations in allele frequencies over time in a manner that is not necessarily important to the biology of the virus. When the alleles that change frequencies are interchangeable in terms of the biology of the organism, such instances of changes are considered neutral evolution. This is especially likely when the number of viruses in a patient is still small. Simply because they are neutral during the period of change in frequencies does not mean that they will always be biologically insignificant. An amino acid substitution in one part of a protein's three-dimensional structure may exist for a long time before it is paired, by chance, with an amino acid substitution in another part of the protein. Without both new amino acids, no new function is expected; however, in patients with both amino acid substitutions, their combined significance may be extremely important. Such paired changes, like any evolutionary outcomes, are difficult to predict.

In viral evolution, the processes of mutation, selection, and chance are all at play. Frequencies of strains can change within a person via competition among strains. They can also change over time, fairly quickly. During transmission, the strain(s) in the highest frequency in the infected person are more likely to be transmitted. When the number of viral particles that are transferred from one person to another is low, chance can play a large role in determining which strain is passed to an individual.

In the landmark *NEJM* study, instances were observed of variants that had low frequencies in early Ebola cases but higher frequencies in later cases. This is evolution, caught red-handed.

In the second case of EVD 2014, Sia had classic hemorrhagic fever, with the tell-tale bleeding. It is possible that early in the transmission of the virus, from Sia to her daughter, or from Emile to his sister, was involved a variant strain that became the predominant strain in Emile's grandmother. Which strain transmitted, and which did not, may have been a determining factor to explain why, this time, we have an epidemic. Luck, in this case bad luck, may be responsible for how widespread this outbreak became via any number of specific mechanisms.

There is scant experimental data on the progression of the disease as the virus courses through the body. We know very little about the effects of Ebola guinea on the physiological workings of the gastrointestinal tract, and how these effects might differ among the various Ebola quasispecies. We will explore a number of possible mechanisms in the next chapter. Without functional studies of various strains, the explorations are speculative, but they are not idle; they are hypotheses that may be important to the defeat of Ebola guinea.

References

Baize *et al.* (2014) Emergence of Zaire ebola virus disease in Guinea. *N Engl J Med* 371: 1418–25. doi: 10.1056/NEJMoa1404505.

Carroll SA, Towner JS, Sealy TK, *et al.* (2013) Molecular evolution of viruses of the family Filoviridae based on 97 whole-genome sequences. *J Virol* **87(5):** 2608–16. doi: 10.1128/JVI.03118-12.

Cite Osterholm on line 6,27 University (Osterholm, 2014).

Formenty P, Leroy EM, Epelboin A, *et al.* (2006) Detection of Ebola virus in oral fluid specimens during outbreaks of Ebola virus hemorrhagic fever in the Republic of Congo. *Clin Infect Dis* **42:** 1521–26.

Gire SK, Goba A, Andersen KG *et al.* (2014) Genomic surveillance elucidates Ebola virus origin and transmission during the 2014 outbreak. *Science* 345(6202): 1369–72. doi: 10.1126/science.1259657.

Goldfrank D, *et al.* (1996) Effect of mammography on breast cancer risk in women with mutations in BRCA1 or BRCA2. *Cancer Epidemiol Biomarker Prev* **15:** 2311–13.

Georges-Courbot MC, Sanchez A, Lu CY, *et al.* (1997) Isolation and phylogenetic characterization of Ebola viruses causing different outbreaks in Gabon. *Emerg Infect Dis* **3(1):** 59–62.

Jaax NK, Davis KJ, Geisbert TJ, *et al.* (1996) Lethal experimental infection of rhesus monkeys with Ebola-Zaire (Mayinga) virus by the oral and conjunctival route of exposure. *Arch Pathol Lab Med* **120:** 140–55.

Jeffers HP. (2014) *Roosevelt the Explorer: T.R.'s Amazing Adventures as a Naturalist, Conservationist, and Explorer.* Taylor Trade Publishing, Rowman & Littlefield, Lanham, MD.

Jordan R, Patel S, Hu H, Lyons-Weiler J. (2008) Efficiency analysis of competing tests for finding differentially expressed genes in lung adenocarcinoma. *Cancer Inform* **6:** 389–421.

Kobinger GP, Leung A, Neufeld J, *et al.* (2011) Replication, pathogenicity, shedding, and transmission of *Zaire ebolavirus* in pigs. *J Infect Dis* **204:** 200–8.

Kortepeter MG, Bausch DG, Bray M. (2011) Basic clinical and laboratory features of filoviral hemorrhagic fever. *J Infect Dis* **204(3):** S810–S816.

Łuksza M, Bedford T, Lässig M. (2014) Epidemiological and evolutionary analysis of the 2014 Ebola virus outbreak. [http://bedford.io/papers/luksza-ebola-evolution/accessed Jan 14, 2015]

Osterholm M. (2014) Challenges for Unprepared Health Systems. Ebola Crisis Deans Symposium, Johns Hopkins University, Oct 14, 2014. [http://www.jhsph.edu/news/special-topics/ebola/ebola-videos/ebola-crisis-deans-symposium-part-6-challenges-for-unprepared-health-systems]

Piercy TJ, Smither SJ, Steward JA, *et al.* (2010) The survival of filoviruses in liquids, on solid substrates and in a dynamic aerosol. *J Appl Microbiol.* **109(5):** 1531–39. doi: 10.1111/j.1365-2672.2010.04778.x.

PRI. (2014) A Liberian describes the hard reality of Ebola: 'You're running even from people you love.' PRI, July 31, 2014. [http://www.pri.org/stories/2014-07-31/liberian-describes-hard-reality-ebola-youre-running-even-people-you-love]

Quammen D. (2014) *Ebola: The Natural and Human History of a Deadly Virus.* WW Norton and Co., New York.

Sefton, Dru. 2014. CDC requests 200 DVDs of Frontline doc to train workers fighting Ebola. Oct Current.org org www.current.org/2014/10/cdc-requests-200-dvds-of-frontline-doc-to-train-workers-fighting-ebola/

Stadler T, Kühnert D, Rasmussen DA, du Plessis L. (2014) Insights into the early epidemic spread of Ebola in Sierra Leone provided by viral sequence data. PLOS Currents: Outbreaks. doi: 10.1371/currents.outbreaks.02bc6d927ecee7bbd33532ec8ba6a25f.1

Twenhafel NA, Shaia CI, Bunton TE, *et al.* (2014) Experimental aerosolized guinea pig-adapted *Zaire ebolavirus* (variant: Mayinga) causes lethal pneumonia in guinea pigs. *Vet Pathol* **52(1):** 21–5. doi: 10.1177/0300985814535612.

Volz E, Pond S. (2014). Phylodynamic analysis of Ebola virus in the 2014 Sierra Leone epidemic. PLOS Currents: Outbreaks. doi: 10.1371/currents.outbreaks.6f7025f1271821d4c815385b08f5f80e.1

Zumbrun EE, Abdeltawab NF, Bloomfield HA, *et al.* (2012) Development of a murine model for aerosolized *ebolavirus* infection using a panel of recombinant inbred mice. *Viruses* **4:** 258–75.

3

Ways in Which Ebola Guinea May Differ from Past Outbreaks: Evolution of Viral Phenotypes

To understand why it is important to consider the genetic variation that does, in fact, exist, and that may distinguish Ebola guinea from previous strains, it is important to understand the ways in which viral biology can change to increase transmissibility. Much of what is described here is based on observations from past outbreaks. These descriptions should not be taken as a fixed understanding of the biology of Ebola guinea.

"Going Airborne"

In the initial weeks of the US press' instant but late infatuation with Ebola in 2014, there was a great deal of discussion on whether the virus had "gone airborne." This almost certainly is a result of that event in the plot development of the 1995 movie *Outbreak*. The initial discussion on Ebola "going airborne" took much-needed attention away from the fact that *Ebolavirus* is a multifaceted organism with numerous characteristics that could change over time, or from patient to patient. The likelihood of Ebola guinea being "airborne" is close to 0%; we would have already seen millions of cases worldwide, with people infecting other people with no direct, casual or indirect contact. But that does not mean that we understand the transmission dynamics.

The term "airborne" is misleading; the more correct process for Ebola is called "aerosolization": spread by nearby transfer of virus borne in droplets of body fluids from one person to another. The most commonly accepted model of aerosolization is due to coughing; an infected patient coughs, or sneezes, and nearby people may then inhale small particles of virus-infected mucous as the primary mode of transmission. This is, in part, why health care workers wear goggles or masks as part of their personal protective gear when interviewing potential EVD patients: In case of accidental discharge. All of the PPG and protection against infection is built on this model.

Hollywood-style "airborne" spread is said to be highly unlikely for this strain; the jury is still out on how efficient transmission is by droplet. In a press conference at the end of July, CDC Director Thomas Frieden initially said:

> *But, remember, Ebola to spread generally requires close contact. It is not spread by the airborne route and it is not spread by someone who is not sick.*

During the Q&A, Rebecca Hamman of the Voice of Nigeria asked:

> *You just said the transmission of Ebola is through close contact. But it seems it's going beyond that. The name itself was derived from a river. Do you mean (that it is) not water-borne or airborne? My people are scared at the rate at which it is being transmitted and moving very fast. I would like to know how Ebola is contracted.*

Dr. Frieden then appeared to backtrack, stating that it has never been proven to be spread by air.

In this thinking, there is a reliance on negative data to make a positive assertion about a knowledge claim, which is not logical. The absence of data for or against a hypothesis does not allow one to accept the null; the only thing that can logically be deduced is that we don't know. Just as it would be wrong to conclude that the virus is airborne, it is incorrect to conclude that this strain has not already acquired, among its many mutations, a new phenotype that makes it more easily aerosolized. If we assume that the mutations that exist do not confer any different functions to the proteins of the virus, then the conclusion would seem warranted. But that's basing a conclusion on an assumption, not on data. The functional studies for the 2014 strains have not been conducted. Studies of the aerosolization of this strain, like those conducted in the past, seem warranted.

Shifting Other Routes of Transmission

A more recently developed transmission concept involves a less restricted model; coughing, sneezing, bleeding, and diarrhea are seen as having something emanating from the patient; the virus is spread around the room in droplets of body fluids, which when dried are called "fomites." These fomites can then be kicked back into the area, carried around on people's clothing and shoes, and be moved around the hospital into non-Ebola wards. If this happens, we can expect health care workers in non-Ebola wards to become infected and sick.

Such is the case of a nurse who worked in the same hospital in Sierra Leone where Dr. Sheik Umar Khan worked in an Ebola ward. Dr. Khan's story is heart-wrenching; he was a rare breed, willing to take the risk necessary to help EVD patients get, and feel better. When diagnosed he removed himself from the ward in which he worked so as to not reduce the morale of his co-workers and he asked to be relocated to a different hospital. A few days after Dr. Khan relocated, the nurse came down with flu-like symptoms; however, she had never even entered the Ebola ward. Here is a description from an article in *The New Yorker* titled "The Ebola Wars":

> *Khan worked long hours in the Ebola wards, trying to reassure patients. Then one of the nurses got sick with Ebola and died. She hadn't even been working in the Ebola ward. The virus particles were*

invisible, and there were astronomical numbers of them in the wards;
they were all over the floor and all over the patients.
(http://www.newyorker.com/magazine/2014/10/27/ebola-wars)

The more complex transmission model is likely the more correct of the two, as it does not rule out passive, indirect transmission over days.

The shock and dismay at the rate of spread of Ebola in 2014 was well deserved. The previous largest outbreak of Ebola was in Uganda, in 2000, killing 425. From the beginning, the question of whether the virus' spread could be attributed to some new biological feature of the virus loomed. *Ebolavirus* can survive outside of the body on various surfaces for varying lengths of time, depending on environmental conditions. One study showed that *Reston ebolavirus* can survive on various surfaces for up to three weeks (Piercy *et al.*, 2010). However, there is also evidence of low transmissibility of the virus via saliva; while viral proteins can exist easily in saliva, RNA cannot. Saliva is a complex mixture of mucous and enzymes, some of which are RNAases, perhaps representing a first line of defense against RNA virus infection.

After reviewing the literature, I find that there is no reason to expect that *Ebolavirus* cannot survive for hours, days and maybe weeks outside the body under certain conditions. Under the right conditions, motes, or specks of dust carrying the virus, can easily be kicked up into the air or transmitted on telephone receivers or common-use devices (Hirsch *et al.*, 2014).

Replicating More Slowly

Patients who die from Ebola infection rarely show the presence of antibodies against the virus. The virus kills most frequently by co-opting the cells in the cardiovascular system for its own reproduction, causing them to become porous, after wreaking havoc on major organs. After initially hiding out in the spleen and liver, the virus moves on to other tissues. The body's cells produce so many viruses so quickly, the blood becomes thick with the virus, organs undergo significant damage, and veins and arteries become porous as the normal processes of coagulation become disrupted. This is not good for the patient, and, in many ways, is not good for the virus. Median survival times of people who die from Ebola are around 6 to 16 days (median usually around nine days after first symptoms), and the patients who die then die fast, very suddenly. Fever in people who will survive lasts around five to nine days. There is ample time for transmission. Just prior to death, the person is transmitting billions of viral particles in sweat, blood, tears, and other body fluids. Some say that Ebola is, in general, hard to catch: At this stage, however, transmission seems very likely. After death, the body is highly contagious; postmortem transmission is therefore a common cause of infection, and thus anything the virus can do to remain active and capable of infecting new people is helpful to the virus.

A longer transmission time could be made possible if the virus were to slow its replication rates so as to make a person sick, but not with life-threatening symptoms. This reduction in virulence is predicted by evolutionary theory of viruses that transfer hosts: A dead host is not good for the virus' longevity. At the end stage of EVD, the virus replicates in an uncontrolled fashion. One way for this virus to become less virulent would be to replicate more slowly and not kill its new host. *Ebolavirus* has already done this, to an extent. The virus uses its membrane-associated protein VP24 to delay the production of interferons (IFNs) and IFN signaling for a while, allow the concentration of virus particles (viremia) to build up to the point of no return, thus become more infectious by escaping immune surveillance long enough to produce transmissible concentrations. If the virus produced too many virions too quickly, the IFNs would have time to work. The virus' subterfuge helps ensure its success.

Asymptomatic Transmission

The oft-stated mantra that one cannot become infected unless one comes into contact with body fluids of a person "sick with

Ebola" represents what is thought to be known about *Ebolavirus*. Barring blood transfusions from an infected person who is not yet symptomatic, the risk of infection is thought to be "so small as to be non-existent" (Dr. Andrew Fauci, NIAID). Transmission from organ transplantation is also a concern, especially due to the virus' likely effect on immunocompromised patients (Kaul *et al.*, 2014).

These statements are relevant for the past strains. An exhaustive independent review of the modes of transmission for all 24 past outbreaks showed no positive claims of asymptomatic transmission (Racaniello, 2014). However, a particularly devilish way in which this virus could increase its transmissibility would be to evolve the ability to be transmitted prior to an infected person showing symptoms, and the statement of no transmission without symptoms is based on past outbreaks. This is the strategy evolved by some of the most successful viruses that spread easily through the human population. These include influenza, the common cold, and viruses that cause so-called stomach flu (gastroenteritis). In some infectious diseases, an infected person is hottest the day before the illness manifests.

The distribution of the number of days after known exposure (assumed incubation period) is telling; while most people show symptoms between 6 and 10 days, a greater than expected percentage of people show symptoms on days 1 and 2 (WHO Ebola Response Team, 2014) beyond that of the lognormal curve fit to the data. That is, days 1 and 2 appear overdispersed in Guinea, Liberia and Sierra Leone. This means there are more cases for those days than expected given the distribution. People tend to see the same people day after day, so a difference of 1 to 2 days might be missed. A simple model that allows a small percentage of asymptomatic transmission a day or two before symptoms could easily accommodate the overdispersion (see WHO Ebola Response Team, 2014, their Fig. 3). It's too early to tell. The right kind of study has yet to be done in non-human primates, where animals are kept side by side in cages with infected animals, with random individuals censored out of the room as the infection develops in the infected monkeys to determine if any exposed only prior to the symptom become infected.

That said, *ebolavirus* even in 2014 is thought to be hard to catch. I was discussing transmission modes with Dr. Gavin MacGregor-Skinner, one of the frontliners in the war in Ebola. He agrees that while microabrasions are a risk, he and his colleagues have direct experience with EVD patients, and even with direct contact, infection is not easy. The patients vomit (some projectile vomit), and the amount of liquid feces produced is, in his words, "incredible, and gets everywhere." In the first two days, he says, all of his patients have diarrhea. As the virus attacks the internal organs in days 4 to 7, they produce more and more, and it turns bloody. As horrific as this sounds, he cited little concern over incidental infection, however, as many times, in spite of precautions, he has experienced getting a patient's feces directly on his skin, at which point his colleagues and he simply wash it off, and they have not been infected. Ebola discoverer Dr. Peter Piot has been quoted as saying he would be comfortable sitting next to a person infected with Ebola on a train "as long as they don't vomit or something" (Smith, 2014). The early stages of vomiting and diarrhea are almost certainly moments of intimate care, and if the fluids are not bloody, it seems that those days may represent a high percentage of instances of infection by loved ones and caregivers.

How would Ebola guinea acquire the ability to become transmissible? One answer is simple: Time. Duration of infection prior to symptoms increases the likelihood of transmission. Every day that an infected asymptomatic person associates with other people increases the possibility, however low, of transmission from a non-infected person. As time goes on, the initially low probability of a single transmission event does not become multiplicatively smaller. Instead, that low probability becomes cumulative (additive) and becomes larger, especially so in a progressing patient. That is, in the context of this epidemic, we're not as interested in the probability that a patient infects at least one person per day; no, that would be a nightmare if those compound probabilities were anything much greater than zero. We're interested in the probability that a given patient will infect more than one patient per the length of the period in which they are capable of passing the virus on.

It is safe to say that the probability of presymptomatic infection, however initially small, increase until logarithmically with viremia in the patient.

In October 2014, NIAID director Anthony Fauci stated in a news interviews that the probability of transmission from an infected person who is not yet showing symptoms is so "diminishingly small as to be non-existent." The probability of a non-symptomatic person who remains asymptomatic infecting a person every day is multiplicative (Monday AND Tuesday AND Wednesday). This is the scenario in which probabilities become "vanishingly small," a phrase that has sometimes been used. However, the probability of such a person infecting ANYONE over the course of a multiple day period is additive for all days: p(Monday) + p(Tuesday) + p(Wednesday)... p(Day X). In this context, the probabilities are cumulative, and are not vanishingly small. As time progresses, infected persons may interact with more people, and the viremia increases in some people day by day. A disease will spread exponentially in a population if an infected person passes the infectious agent, on average, to two or more people. Epidemiologists call this the "transmission rate." Under steady-state transmission, the average transmission rate is 1.0. The disease continues to spread until something changes (like transmission control measures) to cause the average transmission rate to reduce below 1.0. The larger the number of people in the population infected, the greater the probability the disease will be spread. The denser the population, the more likely the virus is to spread to multiple people from one infected person. The number of people who died after become infected from Emile's grandmother's funeral alone was 14.

I checked with an expert in estimating transmission rates, my friend and colleague Dr. Jeffrey Townsend of Yale University, on what the data say. I asked him if it was possible to see, in the transmission data available from the early stages of the outbreak, whether a missing parameter of asymptomatic transmission was needed in his models of estimating transmission rates. His recent study (Scarpino *et al.*, 2014) showed that, over the earliest phase of the outbreak, the percentage of non-reported cases was likely to be

17% of total confirmed cases, far lower than actual cases being 250% of observed cases cited in some "guesstimates." He then pointed out that, at least in the early outbreak in Sierra Leone, it is very unlikely that unreported cases and instances of asymptomatic transmission combined could add up to more than 70% of the number of total confirmed cases.

If the replication rates were shown to be low enough to avoid immune surveillance, but high enough to allow viremia associated with a slightly higher risk of transmission, then Ebola guinea may ultimately be found to have followed the path of other viruses after host transfer to becoming a permanent resident upon humanity.

Change in Host Tissue Virulence Patterns, and Primary Mode of Death

Viruses are not sentient; they are molecular machines that replicate. If Ebola were sentient, it would seem to be making the right decisions about who to infect, and how to affect their bodies in ways that could be most effective at spreading itself to other humans. It can be expected that, after host transfer, viruses will evolve to become less virulent. However, the final story of Ebola's evolution during this outbreak is far from over. One of the most significant factors that can influence the rate of evolution is population size. In an expanding population of Ebola cases, each person represents the equivalent of a newly colonized planet; hundreds of billions of viruses exist in the body, and each time the viral genome replicates, there is a small, but non-zero, probability of a chance mutation. One of these mutations might change the way that virus attacks the immune system. Or, it might change the types of tissues the virus is most likely to infect. It might make the virus capable of hijacking molecular pathways that exist in only a certain type of cell. Any of these types of changes in the viral phenotype could lead to an increase in the number of cases that experience bloody emissis and diarrhea. Avoiding contact with these body fluids, if they occur in high volumes, is very difficult for caregivers.

It seems likely that the evidence accumulated to date would support the hypothesis that one or more of the mutations in the Ebola guinea has led to these types of changes. There is an increase in the percentage of patients who vomit, a decrease in abdominal pain prior to vomiting, and a marked drop in the number of people who exhibit final-stage hemorrhaging. The detailed effects of the different ebolaviruses on various tissues has not yet been thoroughly characterized, but it is also possible that death from dehydration and other events that lead to dark vomit and diarrhea are due to the acquisition of enhanced capabilities to attack the gastrointestinal tract earlier in the course of the disease. Perhaps most Ebola guinea patients who die pass on before the final stage hemorrhaging; that is, no mutation need exist that would prevent bleeding from the eyes, nose, throat and ears. Note that one might predict that the virus may eventually lose its capacity for such a phenotype if it becomes irrelevant to its transmission.

If this thesis is correct, there is a lesson here for other outbreaks and other diseases. The world seemed obsessed for a time on the question of whether *Ebolavirus* had gone "airborne." It seems to be treated as a dichotomous variable; i.e., black and white, yes or no, airborne or not airborne. The nature of evolution by means of natural selection, however, is rarely so clean-cut. If we traced all of our ancestors back 7.5 million years, individual by individual, it would be hard to pinpoint a specific moment in time when modern humans clearly evolved. The same is true with viral phenotypes; at the beginning of the outbreak, there may have been variation among the quasispecies infecting the patients, some of which aggressively attacked the gastrointestinal tract. Over time, those would increase in abundance if they were the type more likely to be transmitted. Thus, dangerous changes in viral phenotypes may be gradual and continuous, and thus hard to detect. We humans like to classify organisms into neat and distinct boxes, when in fact, life is a genetic continuum.

If continuous symptom shift is the case, this means the virus in 2014 is more transmissible due in part to emissis than in prior outbreaks, and that changes in the global response to the Ebola guinea virus should be made based on the expected clinical course of the disease. Quite often in the treatment of EVD patients, they are treated initially for other diseases such as malaria. Part of that treatment is giving fluids; this leads to large volumes of liquid waste. If vomiting and diarrhea could be prevented and the liquid better contained, the disease might spread more slowly. The development and use of technologies that could seal — and immediately neutralize — a person's liquid infectious waste upon exiting could be critical. Perhaps someone could invent a "Tidy Bowl™"-type disinfectant that kills viruses. It would not be difficult.

References

Hirsch EB, Raux BR, Lancaster JW, *et al.* (2014) Surface microbiology of the iPad tablet computer and the potential to serve as a fomite in both inpatient practice settings as well as outside of the hospital environment. *PLOS One.* **9(10):** e111250. Doi: 10.1371/journal. pone.0111250. eCollection 2014.

Kaul DR, Mehta AK, Wolfe CR, *et al.* (2014) Ebola Virus Disease: Implications for Solid Organ Transplantation. *Am J Transplant,* Dec 15, 2014. doi: 10.1111/ajt.13093.

Piercy TJ, Smither SJ, Steward JA, *et al.* (2010) The survival of filoviruses in liquids, on solid substrates and in a dynamic aerosol. *J Appl Microbiol* **109(5):** 1531–9. doi: 10.1111/j.1365-2672.2010.04778.x.

Racaniello V. (2014) Nobel Laureates and Ebola virus quarantine. *Virol Blog,* Nov 4, 2014. [http://www.virology.ws/2014/11/04/nobel-laureates-and-ebola-virus-quarantine/]

Scarpino SV, *et al.,* (2014) Epidemiological and viral genomic sequence analysis of the 2014 Ebola outbreak reveals clustered transmission. *Clin Infect Dis.* doi: 10.1093/cid/ciu1131.

Smith L. 2014. Ebola Discoverer Peter Piot: 'I Would Sit Next to an Infected Person on the Train'. International Business Times, July 31. www.ibtimes.co.uk/ebola-discoverer-peter-piot-i-would-sit-next-infected-person-tube-1459154.

WHO Ebola Response Team. (2014) Ebola Virus Disease in West Africa — The First 9 Months of the Epidemic and Forward Projections. *N Engl J Med* **371:** 1481–95.

4

Biological Knowledge and Ebola Policy

Keeping in mind that this strain seems to move faster, may have a distinct symptomology compared to 2012, has a higher R0, and is, in terms of molecular variation, potentially different in numerous ways than past strains, consider the following:

Ebola is transmitted via direct, or indirect contact with body fluids from an infected person.

That sentence may sound very familiar, but it is different in a very important detail from the often stated mantra of the US Centers for Disease Control and Prevention, which reads that Ebola is spread via:

Direct contact (through broken skin or mucous membranes in, for example, the eyes, nose, or mouth) with

- *blood or body fluids (including but not limited to urine, saliva, sweat, feces, vomit, breast milk, and semen) of a person who is sick with Ebola, and*
- *objects (like needles and syringes) that have been contaminated with the virus*

This has been repeated so often, it is touted as one of the (relatively few) successes in the information campaign by the CDC and the NIH.

However, the key phrase here is *"of a person who is sick with Ebola."* This condition implies a knowledge claim of no latent infectious period for the virus behind the 2014 epidemic.

Note that my phrase reads: "Ebola is transmitted via direct, or indirect contact with body fluids *from an infected person.*"

The difference here is critical: The CDC message, in my view, misleads people to believe that the virus can *never* be spread from an infected person to a non-infected person unless the infected person has symptoms. This is similar to the widely held idea that Ebola cannot travel by airplane. Most people thought that Ebola victims would be too sick to get to the airport. This was proven false via the first ever recorded instance of migration of Ebola via airplane in July 2014 when Patrick Sawyer boarded a plane, bringing Ebola from Monrovia, the capital of Liberia, to Lagos, Nigeria, and again in September 2014 when Thomas Eric Duncan boarded a plane after helping to transport an Ebola patient, bringing *Ebolavirus* to Dallas/Fort Worth. According to a Liberian airport official, Duncan had lied about his history of contact with EVD on an airport questionnaire before boarding a flight to Brussels, where he boarded United Airlines Flight 951 to Washington Dulles International Airport, where he transferred to United Airlines Flight 822 to Dallas/Fort Worth (*New York Times*, Oct 2, 2014).

The idea that no infection is possible before symptoms appear because no recorded cases have proven to involve transmission from asymptomatic infected persons to others is at the core of the CDC's policy making. Its effects can be seen in the willingness of health care workers, who have been exposed, to apparently willfully violate the rules of self-isolation. It is correct to base policy on science; however, it is dangerous to base policy on the unknown. From first principles it can derived that Ebola can be transferred from people who are asymptomatic to others via consideration of receiving a blood transfusion or organ donation from a person suspected of being exposed to *Ebolavirus,* and that a single virion is sufficient, in principle, to cause a fatal infection. Further circumstances would seem to warrant an abundance of caution in policies regarding suspected cases of exposure as well. Consider, for example, thousands of suspected cases wandering freely in a populated city. The probability that a small percentage may turn suddenly sick, in public, does not seem small. The probability that some of those people will experience fairly intimate contact with health care workers for non-Ebola related conditions, such as a broken arm, also does not appear small. If these numbers rise to tens of thousands of suspected exposures, then the low probability of an outbreak becomes a near certainty; some of those people will require blood draws, say, for annual check-ups, or medical care for accidents. They may cut themselves, or be in a car accident, or require stitches, or have a heart attack, requiring intubation. These are the circumstances in which health care workers may be exposed.

In the 1930s, William Wells was studying the modes of transmission of measles and other infectious diseases, and worked out a model of transmission that still impacts our way of thinking. In his model, two major types of dispersal of a pathogen seemed likely. The first of these was transmission via droplets, which was induced by coughing, and sneezing, with droplets traveling to nearby people (within 3–6 feet). The second mode was called airborne, in which the dispersal was achieved via any number of routes of generalized spreading that led to transmission directly through the air in a manner that could impact people at a larger distance. His ideas and the studies that supported them were not easily digested by all of his colleagues, and in a reply to a critique of one of his studies (Wells, 1934), he noted:

Failure to discover air-borne infection ... [doesn't] prove its absence.

The chief policy makers and executors at the CDC and other federal agencies have adamantly and steadfastly insisted that transmission is nearly impossible from asymptomatic infected people. They based this, they say, on years of experience with "this virus" (meaning *Zaire ebolavirus*), and scientific studies that show that high risk of transmission requires high levels of viremia. However, asymptomatic infection has been well documented with both immunoglobulin M (IgM) and G (IgG) responses (Leroy *et al.*, 2000), and is perhaps not uncommon, raising the specter of "carrier"-type transmission.

Wells might have offered advice such as:

Failure to discover presymptomatic transmission of ebolavirus does not prove its absence.

There has been an abundance of reliance on the absence of data as the sole support for positive knowledge claims. We have seen mounting evidence that there may be very important differences between the 2014 strain and strains from past outbreaks. For one:

We are witnessing the world's largest outbreak of Ebolavirus disease in history.

This has been attributed to human factors, such as squalor, poverty, and crowding, which in some places are horrendous. Others point to cultural practices for caring for the dead, and tales of kissing the dead, as if this were somehow an odd practice restricted to communities in West Africa. I recall as a four-year old boy asking if it was okay to kiss my mother goodbye at her funeral. I was allowed. I am grateful for whoever told me it was allowed.

Early in the outbreak, the local conditions and history of the region were seen as contributing factors. Low literacy rates, rare and unsanitary health care settings, lack of running water and electricity, distrust of authorities, especially foreign health care workers, contributed as family member hid their sick loved ones. Other factors include a lack of suitable health care infrastructure: Kono, an eastern district of 350,000 inhabitants in Sierra Leone, had three ambulances when Ebola came calling. Monrovia, the capital of Liberia, had 15 ambulances for 15 million people. The countries were recovering from an upheaval from past civil wars, and the health care infrastructure, particularly in rural areas, was incapable of dealing with this type of challenge.

Certainly some of these factors facilitate the spread of the virus. But the major symptomatic difference that should not be ignored is the sheer volume of infected material produced per patient, which will overwhelm any health care system. This is in comparison to descriptions from the first outbreaks: People lying in pools of their own blood, vomitus, and bloody diarrhea. Some experts see no difference at all between the 2014 clinical symptoms and those of the first outbreaks, including Dr. Peter Piot (Smith, 2014).

Those caring for Thomas Eric Duncan in Texas reported 10 rooms' worth of infected bed sheets and medical waste. In Ebola wards in Western Africa, patients' beds have a hole through which the diarrhea is collected into buckets below. This unsanitary method will ensure splashing and messes that will leave thousands of dried spots, or "motes." The virus can survive outside the body, dried, in dark areas, for days, and in the right conditions, weeks. Health care workers can spread the virus around the hospital to wards involving people that do not treat EVD patients. And, if the idea that some asymptomatic people may be able to spread the disease is correct, the health care workers treating infected patients for non-Ebola symptoms are at risk. As there have never been any studies of the 2014 virus ruling out asymptomatic transmission, the messiness of the disease itself may explain why so many health care workers are becoming infected. But that's merely informed speculation.

Many public health officials and health care workers in the US consider their system so vastly superior to conditions in Africa that they conclude that the outbreak conditions that exist there do not exist here. They can be confident that they will have more options for treating patients, but the viral phenotype of Ebola guinea ensures that it would be a mistake to think that our health care system will ever be truly ready to handle a large outbreak in a major city.

Indirect Transmissions

The CDC Website also includes the statement:

> *Ebola is spread through direct contact… with objects (like needles and syringes) that have been contaminated with the virus.*

There are additional objects that seem important to consider. The question of whether one could become infected, such as via shared towels (as in methicillin-resistant *Staphylococcus aureus* (MRSA) transmission), or shared toothbrushes and dentist drills (as in HIV transmission) is unanswered. Little is known about the fate of *Ebolavirus* released into modern sewage systems.

The *Ebolavirus* is known to be in high concentrations in saliva at the earliest stages of the disease. It would be safest to assume that someone who has flu symptoms may transmit the disease to loved ones via indirect transmission.

MRSA Indirect Transmission Analogy

Methicillin-resistant *Staphylococcus aureus* is a disease of recent note in the US and elsewhere. *Staphylococcus aureus* in a common bacterial infection usually treatable by antibiotics. During the 1940s and 1950s, widespread use of antibiotics to treat a variety of types of microbes led to the evolution of resistance within *Staphylococcus aureus*. The introduction of Methicillin in 1959 led to the discovery of Methicillin-resistant *Staphylococcus aureus* in 1961 (Enright *et al.*, 2002). This is just about 50 years ago, around the time of the estimated origin of the species *Zaire ebolavirus*.

The number of incidental MRSA infections that occur due to indirect infections in the US per year is estimated at over 79,000 patients per year. The durability of MRSA on fomites can be as high as eight weeks (Desai *et al.*, 2011).

According to the Material Safety Data Sheet (MSDS) on Ebola:

SURVIVAL OUTSIDE HOST: The virus can survive in liquid or dried material for a number of days. Infectivity is found to be stable at room temperature or at 4°C for several days, and indefinitely stable at −70°C (6, 20). Infectivity can be preserved by lyophilisation.

(http://www.msdsonline.com/resources/msds-resources/
free-safety-data-sheet-index/ebola-virus.aspx)

And from the Canadian Pathogen Safety Data Sheet:

SURVIVAL OUTSIDE HOST: Filoviruses have been reported capable to survive for weeks in blood and can also survive on contaminated surfaces, particularly at low temperatures (4°C). One study could not recover any Ebolavirus from experimentally contaminated surfaces (plastic, metal or glass) at room temperature. In another study, Ebolavirus dried onto glass, polymeric silicone rubber, or painted aluminum alloy is able to survive in the dark for several hours under ambient conditions (between 20°C and 25°C and 30–40% relative humidity) (amount of virus reduced to 37% after 15.4 hours), but is less stable than some other viral hemorrhagic fevers (Lassa). When dried in tissue culture media onto glass and stored at 4°C, Zaire ebolavirus survived for over 50 days. This information is based on experimental findings only and not based on observations in nature. This information is intended to be used to support local risk assessments in a laboratory setting.

http://www.phac-aspc.gc.ca/lab-bio/res/psds-ftss/ebola-eng.php

From these sources, *Ebolavirus* seems more durable than the "few hours" given it by the CDC. If indirect MRSA transmission leads to over 70,000 cases per year, and the virus can survive eight weeks on surfaces outside of the body, the number of indirect transmission cases expected per year for *Ebolavirus* is, for various estimates:

Fomite	Time	Expected # of Transmissions/Yr
Surface	"days" (assume 3)	3,750
Blood	"weeks" (assume 2)	17,500
Dried on glass	50 days	62,500

It seems highly unlikely that the intent of the statements of "low indirect transmission" is to facilitate 3,750 to 17,500 Ebola transmissions in the US per year. The question of whether MRSA transmission rates provide a good model for Ebola is an important one. Data on the indirect spread of *Ebolavirus* are scarce; however, the published data do not match the public statements that *Ebolavirus* can only last outside of the body for "minutes, a few hours at most." In one study, a small percentage, but some *Ebolavirus* virions of the Zaire strain were found to be biologically active after 8 hours to direct ultraviolet (UV), mimicking sunlight (Sagripanti *et al.* (2010)). In the same study, virions of *Zaire ebolavirus* kept in the dark were found to last as long as six *days*. At low temperatures on glass slides, *Ebolavirus* has been found to last six weeks (Piercy *et al.*, 2010). Studies of the persistence of *Ebolavirus* on various surfaces such as linens, hospital curtains, bed rails and other places have not been conducted.

Another concern is the disposal of the liquid waste. Looking at other model organisms that cause gastroenteritis, Bibby *et al.* (2014) drew the following conclusions from analysis of the available published data:

> *The available evidence suggests that Ebola virus is inactivated at a rate more rapid than or comparable to those of typically monitored enteric viruses. Additionally, while environmental exposure is not the dominant exposure route, available data suggest that it is imprudent to dismiss the potential of environmental transmission without further evidence.*

He and his colleagues had compared survival of *Ebolavirus* over time in guinea pig sera and compared them to published die-off data of various model human pathogens in tap water. *Ebolavirus* fell right in the middle of persistence, with some *Ebolavirus* remaining viable even after 30 days (Fig. 4.1).

I called Kyle Bibby, a researcher at the University of Pittsburgh, to inquire further on his thoughts. He told me that the current standard of disposal, from the WHO and the CDC, is "down the drain." He is concerned: *"We're told that it's inactivated in minutes in water. There are no data to substantiate that claim. We don't*

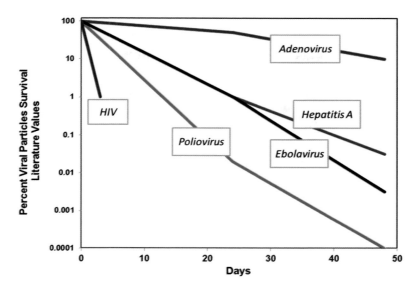

Fig. 4.1 Survival of various viral pathogens as reported in studies compiled by Bibby *et al.* (2014). *Ebolavirus* and HIV were studied in cell culture media; all others were as reported in tap water. Data kindly provided for figure by Kyle Bibby. Data compiled from sources within Bibby *et al.* (2014).

know, for example, if the virus remains viable when it's disposed of that way." He said the primary concern would be workers who would have to come into contact with this waste.

In a densely populated residential area, waste disposal of 3–4 gallons per patient per day could even, perhaps, make the sewer systems a potential ecosystem that could harbor the virus indefinitely. The risk of possible new vector transmission from animals in the sewage systems should be studied.

Dr. Bibby is studying, with a grant from the National Science Foundation, possible surrogate model organisms for studies focused on aerosolization of *Ebolavirus* from toilets. Additional types of studies that Dr. Bibby would like to see done include a study of the microbial organisms in the waste water of developed areas of Monrovia. "*Live culture studies can be limited for environmental studies,"* he said. *"We need to do a PCR-based metagenomics study and find out."*

The CDC also has an infographic that contains the statement: *"You CAN'T get Ebola through FOOD grown or legally purchased in the U.S."* (emphasis theirs). The infographic appears to ignore this observation made in 2007 by the authors of a study published in the *Journal of Infectious Diseases* (Bausch *et al.*, 2007):

> *Of particular concern is the frequent presence of EBOV in saliva early during the course of disease, where it could be transmitted to others through intimate contact and from sharing food, especially given the custom, in many parts of Africa, of eating with the hands from a common plate.*

Doctors and Nurses, The First Line of Defense

The health care workers fighting EVD in Africa risk their lives to help turn the tide. They are forced to witness gruesome deaths, and have to deal with the aftermath. They deserve our upmost respect.

Ebolavirus is listed as a US Federal Select Agent (see www. selectagents.gov). As such, it is subject to Select Agent Regulations. *Ebolaviruses* and Marburg viruses are classified as Category A bio-terrorism agents in the US, and have the potential to pose a risk to national security. Regulation of the movement of the virus is taken very seriously. Some health care workers in the US who are under a 21-day watch period seem bent on violating the rules of self-monitoring and controlled movement. People who have traveled to countries with outbraks are advised to report their daily tempera-ture daily, and the presence or absence of other EVD symptoms (headache, joint and muscle aches, weakness, diarrhea, vomiting, stomach pain, lack of appetite, or abnormal bleeding). They are also required to report their intent to travel in-state or out-of-state, and avoid public transportation. Controlled movement means (a) avoid crowded places, and (b) no use of public transport. Many in the US were dismayed by the news of the behavior of Dr. Spencer, who upon returning from Guinea to New York City, went bowling, rode the subway, and went to dinner — knowing he could potentially fall sick at any time and become infectious. According to the WHO, Dr. Spencer should have:

1. Checked his temperature twice daily
2. Finished a course of malaria prophylaxis (to avoid confusion of Ebola with Malaria)
3. Mastered the relevant symptoms, such as fever;
4. Stayed within four hours of a hospital with isolation facilities;
5. Immediately contacted the MSF-USA office if any relevant symptoms developed.

Considering these criteria, Dr. Spencer did nothing wrong. But the question of the possibility of a sudden onset of illness in a crowded area causes concern over these criteria.

People were equally puzzled, and concerned, by the news that one nurse was given approval by the CDC to board an airplane and travel from Ohio back to Texas in spite of having a symptom (fever of 100.4°) and in spite of being under controlled travel orders. CDC Director Thomas Frieden admitted that she should not have been given the approval to travel. She and her colleagues were exposed to potential infection by *Ebolavirus* as they treated Mr. Duncan. At the time, the CDC website had the wrong PPE; instead of the correct BSL4 protective gear, they had general PPE, which left skin exposed. Their method of glove removal was wrong for Ebola as well. Use of general PPE could lead to what medical practitioners call "self-exposure," increasing the likelihood of infection via the process of taking off the PPE. The CDC quickly removed the incorrect webpage for a while, until they could develop the correct graphic for PPE for EVD. It is worth noting, that the CDC's requirements for respiratory protections for EVD exceed those of the WHO (Michael Osterholm, *pers. comm. to pers. comm.*).

Media uproar ensued when another nurse, who showed a fever upon her return from Sierra Leone, announced that she would refuse to abide by the state of Maine's 21-day quarantine, and then threatened to sue the State of Maine if they attempted to

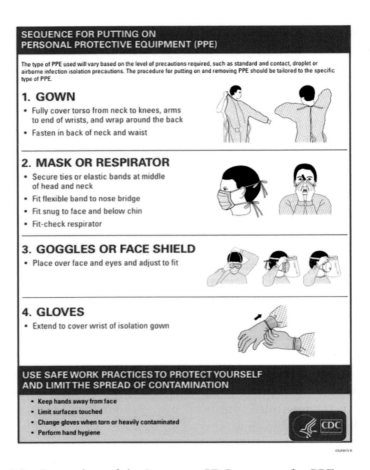

Fig. 4.2 Screenshot of the incorrect CDC resource for PPE use when caring for EVD patients on Oct 15, 2014. This error was pointed out by many medical experts in the Twittersphere. No skin should be showing, and the facial coverage is insufficient. Dr. Frieden defended this information to Megan Kelly on *Fox News*, stating: "Our information is clear, and correct," and was criticized for appearing to blame the infected nurses by citing a "breach of protocol" that must have happened leading to their exposure and infection. In late December, a case of EVD was diagnosed in Edinburgh, Scotland. Photos of health care workers training for use of PPE showed this incorrect type of gear. See Wichmann *et al.* (2014) for an independent, correct description of necessary PPEs.

quarantine her. This nurse was asymptomatic and never tested positive for *Ebolavirus.* She justified her behavior as necessary to prevent health care workers returning from Africa from having to suffer from time off work simply because they might be infected with *Ebolavirus.* She shared her feelings in an essay written for the *Dallas Morning News*:

> *I am scared about how health-care workers will be treated at airports when they declare that they have been fighting Ebola in West Africa... I am scared that, like me, they will arrive and see a frenzy of disorganization, fear and, most frightening, quarantine.*

Her sentiments were echoed by NIH Director Anthony Fauci. In an interview with *ABC News,* he said:

> *We have to be careful when we make policy, that we don't have unintended consequences... I'm concerned of the disincentive for the health care workers.*

Maine Governor Paul LePage sought a court order for judicial validation of the quarantine; the court came down in the middle, refusing to allow outright quarantine, but requiring the nurse to provide daily medical updates and inform the state of any planned travel.

In contrast to civilian protocols, Major General James Lariviere told the US House Oversight Committee that the US military (specifically, the Department of the Army) requires that all civilians contractors in West African countries stay a minimum of three feet away from all US military personnel in the field tending to the building of the infrastructure needed to isolate the growing numbers of EVD patients. Military personnel returning from building treatment centers are also quarantined for 21 days up on their return to the US or before being returned to deployment. These soldiers were being held in Italy, the US, and the Philippines.

After these events, the CDC updated their guidance on travel, and decided to create categories into which they would classify people according to levels of risk (CDC, 2014). For asymptomatic individuals in the High Risk Category, into which all health care workers with direct care experience of EVD patients fall:

> *Controlled movement limits the movement of people. For individuals subject to controlled movement, travel by long-distance commercial conveyances (e.g., aircraft, ship, bus, train) should not be allowed. If travel is allowed, it should be by noncommercial conveyance such as private chartered flight or private vehicle and occur with arrangements for uninterrupted active monitoring. Federal public health travel restrictions (Do Not Board) may be used to enforce controlled movement. For people subject to controlled movement, use of local public transportation (e.g., bus, subway) should be discussed with and only occur with approval of the local public health authority.*

> — Interim US Guidance for Monitoring and Movement of
> Persons with Potential Ebola Virus Exposure
> (Updated again Nov 28, 2014)

There are two points of view here; in the first, the paramount importance is to reduce the spread of infection of Ebola in Western African countries, because the epidemiological models predict an increased likelihood of pandemic. The second point of view is that held by Governor Cuomo of New York, and Governor Christie of New Jersey: They see it as their duty to protect their populations.

The rights of the individual vs. the rights of the many are in balance if the individual acts in a manner that is consistent with the protection of the rights of the many, and vice versa. In the case of EVD, there is a 21-day gap in the clinical community's ability to diagnose the disease. Options for testing currently include antibody-capture enzyme-linked immunosorbent assay (ELISA), antigen detection tests, serum neutralization tests, reverse transcriptase polymerase chain reaction (RT-PCR) assay, electron microscopy and virus isolation by cell culture.

None of the 80 or so tests for point-of-care testing or diagnostic testing currently under consideration by the WHO is capable of reliably detecting the virus in presymptomatic persons. As a result, a negative result during the active and direct monitoring period is currently only useful if it is positive. Thus, the individuals who may have been exposed to *Ebolavirus* are in a medical, and legal, no-man's land. There are many who are concerned that the CDC had to update their guidances in direct response to public concerns over exposure to *Ebolavirus* in health care workers returning from Western African countries.

Another concern is fairly practical: The effects of three week's isolation on the finances of those who fall under the guidelines. The State of New Jersey has implemented a plan to pay lost wages to people under state-imposed restrictions. Another possibility is that employers work with insurance companies to work out the terms of Quarantine Insurance, allowing people to use it like unemployment insurance if they fall into circumstances where they need to be isolated to protect the population.

The media coverage of the first cases of EVD in the US can only be described as "frantic." That said, they did not know, and, I submit, we still do not know, the ultimate endpoint for this epidemic. During those weeks, any suspected case of EVD was given a thorough treatment. In October, the White House requested what they characterized as more responsible reporting. In a blog statement, the AP reported that they would keep their stories covering suspected EVD "brief, and in perspective" (AP, 10/17/2014). Was this censorship? What amounts to a fair balance of the public's right to know that their neighbor may be infected with *Ebolavirus,* and the individual's right to privacy? The American public should be better educated when the topic is a highly infectious agent. On Ebola, the press should be responsible in their reporting, and help spread the news that negative tests before the 21 day period has ended should be interpreted as "inconclusive."

At the time of this writing (December 2014), "active post-arrival monitoring" is the norm for people returning to New York, Pennsylvania, Maryland, Virginia, New Jersey, and Georgia from (directly or indirectly) Liberia, Sierra Leone, or Guinea.

The situation in the UK is not much better than in the US. In late December 2014, a Scottish nurse returning from Sierra Leone, where she had cared for EVD patients, tested positive. Upon her team's return from Africa, the scene at the airport was described as a "reunion," with close personal contact (hugging, kissing). The nurse was asymptomatic at the airport. A doctor who sat next to the nurse roundly criticized Public Health England for what he described as "bizarre" quarantine policies. At the time, individuals traveling from countries with EVD were expected to make their way home using public transport, but only using any particular shared vehicle for an hour at time. Then, once home, they were asked to eschew public transportation of any kind. A person's decision to take a single train home could, in principle, be not recommended while his or her decision to take the train for one hour, potentially exposing train-goers, then wait in a bus station and take a bus, exposing more, then maybe share a cab, would be better recommendations.

Reverse White Coat Syndrome?

The US medical system does not tend to see itself in any way as a possible source of disease for its patients; again, this goes against many peer-reviewed published studies that have shown health care worker to patient transmission of everything from HIV (Bosch, 2003) to Hepatitis B (Buster *et al.*, 2003). Even iPad tablet computers have been shown to act as reservoirs of dangerous pathogens in the hospital setting (Hirsch *et al.*, 2014). Consider that, for correct and ethical reasons, the number of controlled clinical trials studying the transmission of *Ebolavirus* in asymptomatic infected persons to others in humans is 0.

Available data seem to indicate that more people are vomiting, and fewer people are experiencing abdominal pain and bleeding with this Ebola from Guinea (2014) than from the Ebola in Zaire (2012).

There is an unusually high percentage of health care worker deaths due to Ebola infection in Western African countries.

The health care workers infected in the US during their treatment of Thomas Eric Duncan, and the nurse in Spain all said that they followed protocols, and said had no idea how they become infected. A nurse who had never worked in an Ebola ward, and who worked with Dr. Khan, got sick with Ebola and died.

CDC Director Thomas Frieden's testimony that there are no mutations in the 2014 strain, when in fact there are nearly 400 mutations, many of which change the sequence of the viral proteins, seems inconceivable.

I found myself confused. For a few months, when both Ebola and fear circulated on US soil, there was a great deal of conflicting information. Time and again I found Dr. Gavin MacGregor-Skinner to be one of the most passionate voices for reason on the air at the time. He appeared in interview after interview on *CNN*, *CNBC*, the *BBC* and other news television channels spreading the word not about how bad EVD is, but rather, what shortcomings exist in our institutions, our policies and our practices, and how they could be fixed. In writing this book, I knew I needed to speak with Gavin. Early one morning in December, after dropping my sons off at school, I called Gavin. We discussed Ebola for about an hour and a half. I was curious about his perspective on things now that the hysteria had died down, and we had some time to reflect. In a nutshell, Gavin's messages were consistent with those he presented during those earlier odd months: The emergency response systems in the US are not structured correctly, and we are not using all the tools we have in the toolbox.

At the hospital level, in Texas, Gavin feels there were lessons to be learned that he is afraid might be missed. He was concerned that the existing hierarchy within the hospital was used to respond to the Ebola case. "There was not a ready-made separate management and supervision procedure in place for BSL4 agent where a 25-year-old nurse could tell a 55-year-old doctor to stop doing what he's doing due to a protocol breach." Gavin told me: *"Instead, the existing hospital administrative hierarchy was used, and they were not trained, not anywhere near ready."* He noted that the Occupational Health and Safety Administration also did not conduct an investigation. *"OSHA's involved on a routine basis all of the time, for even a single needle prick. Where was OSHA?"* I knew I was speaking to the same passionate Gavin.

Gavin's concerns about the process only begin at the local level. "No one," he said, "invoked ESF8." ESF8 is a national emergency response plan. If it had been activated, it would have brought resources to bear on the problem. Instead of using the emergency response system in place, we froze for fear of making a big deal out of nothing. Said Gavin: *"Risk is still a four-letter word in the United States."* While there is a Hospital Infection Control program in place in most US hospitals, for him these programs place too much emphasis on control and accountability, which are in many ways reactive activities, instead of proactive behaviors that initiate as planned crisis response.

Infection control is not the correct process, according to Gavin, and it should be replaced by a Biorisk Management System. I was floored to learn during our discussion that The World Health Organization published a manual for emergency response to these types of agents, but, according to Gavin: "No one read it."

I asked for a good example of a ready-made response. He had one. Everyone should compare and contrast the readiness and response of the US to Ebola to that of the Health and Human Services Pandemic Influenza Plan, which Gavin described as an "in place, proactive plan of action that was activated upon the emergence of the disease." This is the type of system by which Texas could have had a ready-made, drilled, practiced, accredited response team on site who knew how to respond to the first diagnosis of EVD with checklists and SOPs. This approach, he said, builds confidence and directs human behavior in a setting where what people do can determine whether the virus spreads or not. The existing system was ill-prepared to attempt to handle the case without outside help. No readiness program existed in Texas. The CDC has also been criticized by some for not having arrived right away to help. Instead, hospital staff had to handle the situation on their own, being referred to the CDC website for training, a website which contained incorrect information on which person protective equipment health care workers should use.

They, and everyone else it seems, were not prepared. At the time of the Duncan case, there were five beds in the US capable of being used to adequately treat patients infected with BSL4 infectious agents, and the CDC website's material for protective gear showed the wrong PPE gear. Someone had used the image of the gear for influenza. The Departments of Public Health at the State level, said Gavin, are the champions of the need for changes such as a regionalization of information transfer and coordination of treatment centers. In early December, the CDC announced the creation of 35 hospitals; however, they need to be accredited, and no SOPs or ISOs yet exist by which they can be evaluated, by checklist, on an annual basis, for Ebola readiness. Gavin's perspective is that the US model may be stretched too thin: The maintenance cost of Ebola readiness at 35 hospitals, supporting 52 beds, is inferior, he thinks, to the Nigerian model of two dedicated hospitals, with over 70 beds combined. This would minimize the geographic risk and help contain the spread out from the hospitals to the community.

Gavin is not alone in thinking that the existing infrastructure is not matched to the task of tackling a widespread outbreak of a highly infectious disease. Others also envision an Emergency Management System, hierarchically located above the CDC, the NIH, HS, HHS, and FEMA, focused on logistics, communication, information sharing, supplies and allocation of resources. The CDC, he said, is very good at what they are trained to do: Shutting down epidemics with contact tracing. No one there, he said, is trained in logistics, and they were left to do what they could do without formal training.

Policy should be the expression of actionable knowledge, grounded in solid knowledge. This knowledge can be hard to come by, and the time to generate it is not during a crisis, but beforehand. The US effectively had no plan for health care workers potentially exposed to a biological agent abroad during their service.

Each person had to learn of their responsibilities anew. I asked Gavin if he knew who could have activated ESF8? "It takes a disaster declaration," he said. I wondered if he had any idea as to how many cases of Ebola would have been a reasonable cut-off before ESF8 activation. "That's a good question," was Gavin's reply.

There is currently draft legislation in the works to improve emergency preparedness in response to a biological crisis. Gavin is concerned that any such initiatives would have to be able to be structured to "maintain capabilities of responsiveness." *"It's paying for the maintenance of readiness that concern me,"* he said, *"during the down times, when there is no crisis. There's got to be drilling, and annual accreditation, and site visits, and check lists. It's too easy to make mistakes in readiness."*

The public remains concerned that self-monitoring may be insufficient and that it may be a recipe for an eventual outbreak in the US. New Jersey Governor Chris Christie's sentiment was revealed on *Fox News Sunday*: *"I don't think when you're dealing with something as serious as this you can count on a voluntary system. This is the government's job."*

This perspective is often represented as "fear-mongering." However, science may be in support of the notion that a surprising percentage of health-care workers may not be faithful to the rules of self-monitoring.

A study in Infection Control and Hospital Epidemiology in 2009 (Rao *et al.*, 2009) supports the concern that people will not adhere to self-quarantine conditions. In the study, 102 staff members were asked to endure self-quarantine while infected with norovirus violated the social distancing recommendations:

> *A large norovirus outbreak affecting hospital patients and staff occurred during the winter of 2007. We administered a survey to affected staff to evaluate adherence to social distancing recommendations. Of the 102 survey respondents, 74 (73%) completed self-quarantine. Staff adherence was similar regardless of job responsibility. Incomplete adherence to recommendations could potentially accelerate and prolong infectious disease outbreaks.*

Twenty-seven percent of people in the study violated their self-monitored quarantine. This means up to a full 27% (over one-quarter) of people trusted with their own quarantine can be expected to willfully place others at risk of developing intestinal gastroenteritis caused by norovirus due to their decisions and behaviors. Each individual's motives for violating the recommendations may be unique, but this behavior has one effect on public health: It increases the risk of spreading the disease, regardless of the intent of the person being monitored. Such risk tolerances may be demotivated by monetary reward. Given the immense cost of treating EVD, and other highly infectious diseases, a quarantine insurance model may be a good route to consider.

For some experts, like Dr. Michael Osterholm, the comparison to norovirus has little relevance. He believes that because early interventions have such a profound effect on outcome with EVD, self-monitoring and health status reporting is in such high interest to the individual that virtually every health care worker can be expected to report. I asked him whether he thought health care workers should be isolated upon their return from areas with EVD. He said:

> *There should be a requirement of professional distancing, for sure. Imagine a health care worker who had just worked for five days on patients coming down with this. The effects that it would have on the institution would be overwhelming, even if no transmissions had occurred. No health care worker would want to bring that down on their institution, or to put patients at risk. But do I think they should be totally isolated from society? Absolutely not.*

The perspective that individuals might not be trusted with their own restrictions might be more understandable if the CDC had appeared better organized in their initial response with orderly protocols; if the CDC had not reported, there were no new mutations in this strain; if, as the CDC reported, we actually knew this virus. But there are mutations, plenty of them, and in many ways, despite reassurances, we do not really know this 2014 strain as well as might be hoped. Instead, there is ample evidence that there is something different with this strain of *Ebolavirus* from Guinea. Each new infection, each new death, is another bit of evidence in favor of there perhaps being something amiss with our understanding of this wee beastie, and our current approaches to controlling the outbreak may be missing their mark.

It's time to turn to science, and to start constructing hypotheses of transmission that may or may not include consideration of whether the virus has become more easily transmitted. For example: What effects, if any, do the amino acid substitutions found in the Ebola guinea strain so far have on the virus' phenotype? Do any of them make ribosomal slippage more, or less likely? Do any affect the replication rates within cells? Do any of the mutations confer an earlier preference for gastrointestinal lining? Can any of these changes explain the low rates of abdominal pain? Do any appear to be associated with high numbers of transmission events per unit time? How complete is our understanding of the transmission dynamics of Ebola? Given the immense concentration of virus in body fluids from people sick with Ebola, could our health care system be overwhelmed by even a few hundred cases in the US?

Could asymptomatic infected patients being treated for non-Ebola related medical conditions also be infecting health care workers? Could asymptomatic health care workers be infecting patients, and each other?

A recent study in Liberia seems to confirm that missed recognition of EVD is an important factor and mode of transmission (Matanock *et al.*, 2014), and concludes that infection control measures are needed even in non-Ebola treatment health centers:

West Africa is experiencing the largest Ebola virus disease (Ebola) epidemic in recorded history. Health care workers (HCWs) are at increased risk for Ebola. In Liberia, as of August 14, 2014, a total of 810 cases of Ebola had been reported, including 10 clusters of Ebola cases among HCWs working in facilities that were not Ebola treatment units (non-ETUs). The Liberian Ministry of Health and

Social Welfare and CDC investigated these clusters by reviewing surveillance data, interviewing county health officials, HCWs, and contact tracers, and visiting health care facilities. Ninety-seven cases of Ebola (12% of the estimated total) were identified among HCWs; 62 HCW cases (64%) were part of 10 distinct clusters in non-ETU health care facilities, primarily hospitals. Early recognition and diagnosis of Ebola in patients who were the likely source of introduction to the HCWs (i.e., source patients) was missed in four clusters. Inconsistent recognition and triage of cases of Ebola, overcrowding, limitations in layout of physical spaces, lack of training in the use of and adequate supply of personal protective equipment (PPE), and limited supervision to ensure consistent adherence to infection control practices all were observed. Improving infection control infrastructure in non-ETUs is essential for protecting HCWs. Since August, the Liberian Ministry of Health and Social Welfare with a consortium of partners have undertaken collaborative efforts to strengthen infection control infrastructure in non-ETU health facilities.

One sign of asymptomatic transmission would be the development of antibodies to *Ebolavirus* in people who never developed symptoms, such as was found in health care workers treating SARS patients in Singapore (Wilder-Smith *et al.*, 2005). Past findings of antibodies to *Ebolavirus* and Marburg virus in never-symptomatic persons in African countries has always been attributed to past exposures; if *Ebolavirus* antibodies start showing up in the US in asymptomatic people, we have to assume that they may be capable of transferring the virus to others.

A report issued in December 2014 by the WHO estimated that the risk of a health care worker becoming infected was 100 times that of the normal population in Sierra Leone. Dr. Brima Kargbo, Sierra Leone's chief medical officer, was quoted as saying he was "baffled" by the results of a CDC report (Kilmarx *et al.*, 2014) in which it was reported that as many as 70% of infections in health care workers did not come from Ebola holding centers or treatment facilities (Voice of America, *Sierra Leone Baffled by Doctors'*

Ebola Deaths, Aug 12, 2014.). The increased rate of transmission, and the consistently higher pattern of infections to health care workers, has been attributed to health care workers caring for friends, neighbors and families outside of treatment centers, and to the fact that some patients are not honest about their contact with EVD patients.

There are also large numbers of patients who report no exposure to symptomatic persons. The patient who brought Ebola from Monrovia to Nigeria reported that he had no idea how he contracted the disease. He said that he had never been in contact with anyone with the illness, meaning he potentially acquired the infection from an asymptomatic person (Shaib *et al.*, 2014). Then there is the case of asymptomatic transmission that appeared to have occurred in Sierra Leone. A report indicated that a baby who was asymptomatic and tested negative transmitted the disease to 13 nurses; 12 of the 13 nurses who held the baby contracted EVD ("When Holding An Orphaned Baby Can Mean Contracting Ebola." *NPR Morning Edition*, Oct 10, 2014.) Sadly, it was reported that the nurses all knew the baby likely had the disease. The fact that a negative test is meaningless must be better appreciated.

The best way to determine if EVD is being spread due to asymptomatic transmission is molecular epidemiology: The chain of mutations in the lineages should show instances of transmission from people who did not have symptoms at the time when contact would have taken place. Therefore, securing samples from patients should become a high priority for cases of known and uncertain origin to allow rapid assignment of cases to particular transmission chains. Interview data should be collected on the question: "Have you been in contact with anyone who did not have Ebola symptoms at the time of contact, but who then went on to develop EVD?" We cannot answer the question of asymptomatic transmission unless the data are collected.

It has been speculated that the methods intended to protect health care workers could somehow be making exposure more likely. Consider the testimony from Dr. Beth Bell (Director, National Center for Emerging and Zoonotic Infectious Diseases,

Centers for Disease Control and Prevention) in the US Senate Appropriations Hearings in September 2014:

> *We would not be seeing infections in health care workers if our infection control measures are working.*

The training is short-term; the supplies are low, yes, the health care systems are collapsing. Yes, there are human factors. But what about the virus? Has it acquired a characteristic that happens to allow it to circumvent the control measures?

Could the virus, like rabies, alter reasoning centers of the brain, causing people to think or behave in ways that might make transmission more likely? Could the virus change the drive of people to associate (their sociality), making transmission more likely? Objective, properly observational controlled before-and-after personality surveys could help answer questions like this.

There is some evidence that viruses can affect the hosts' cognitive processes. This is not too far-fetched; one of the symptoms of Marburg virus disease is aggression. If the virus could make people less agreeable to authority, or, in some way, more social (driven to be near people), it could be more readily transmissible. Alteration of host behavior is seen in rabies virus infection in mammals (including humans) and in parvovirus infection in dogs. Some species of tropical ants (Mongkolsamrit *et al.*, 2014) and other insects (Eberhard *et al.*, 2014) infected with fungal spores climb plants and implant their mandibles in the stem and stay there until they die. The fungal body then grows out of their carcasses, and the spores seek other insects. Borna viruses are known to cause self-destructive behaviors in horses (mortality 80–100%), and have been shown to alter social behaviors in rats. The expression of their RNAs has, controversially, been associated with psychotic disorder in humans (Miranda *et al.*, 2006). They have been shown to be incorporated into the genomes of mammalians (Horie *et al.*, 2010) and of invertebrates (Horie *et al.*, 2013).

Other examples of organisms influencing human behaviors have been noted; the existence of a chlorovirus in throat cultures of human subjects was found to reduce their ability to perform on cognitive tests of visual processing and visual motor speed by 10% (Yolken *et al.*, 2014). No studies to date have been conducted on the possible effects of *Ebolavirus* on behavior in humans. Confusion, irritability, and aggression are symptoms of Marburg hemorrhagic fever (WHO Marburg hemorrhagic fever fact sheet, Global Alert and Response, March 31, 2005); the Marburg virus is a close relative of *Ebolavirus*.

Has the *Ebolavirus* shifted in 2014 to become a disease more like cholera and dysentery, and less like a hemorrhagic fever? Are there behavioral differences that might aid the spread? The evidence to date is suggestive; however, more systematic data collection on symptoms is needed. Is the 2014 virus an old strain, just now finding its way into the human population, with different effects on humans than strains from earlier outbreaks? These questions deserve immediate close scrutiny with exacting, hypothesis-based, properly controlled (using correct comparison groups, to avoid bias), and sufficiently powered (large enough sample sizes) scientific studies, including cell culture studies, animal studies and response adaptive randomized clinical trials for treatments. There is a diversity of robust study design types that can be used to effectively address these, and related important questions.

References

AP. (2014) Advisory on Ebola coverage. [http://blog.ap.org/2014/10/17/advisory-on-ebola-coverage/]

Bausch DG, Towner JS, Dowell SF (2007) Assessment of the risk of Ebola virus transmission from bodily fluids and fomites. *J Infect Dis* **196(2):** S142–47.

Bibby K, Casson LW, Stachler E, Haas CN. (2014) Ebola virus persistence in the environment: state of the knowledge and research needs. *Environ Scie Technol Lett* 141209010011006. doi: 10.1021/ez5003715. [http://pubs.acs.org/doi/abs/10.1021/ez5003715]

Bosch X. (2003) Second case of doctor-to-patient HIV transmission. *Lancet Infect Dis* **3(5):** 261.

Buster EH, van der Eijk AA, Schalm SW. (2003) Doctor to patient transmission of hepatitis B virus: Implications of HBV DNA levels and potential new solutions. *Antiviral Res* **60(2):** 79–85.

CDC. (2014) Epidemiologic risk factors to consider when evaluating a person for exposure to Ebola virus. [www.cdc.gov/vhf/ebola/exposure/risk-factors-when-evaluating-person-for-exposure.html]

Desai R, Pannaraj PS, Agopian J, *et al.* (2011) Survival and transmission of community-associated methicillin-resistant Staphylococcus aureus from fomites. *Am J Infect Control* **39(3):** 219–225. doi: 10.1016/j.ajic.2010.07.005.

Eberhard W, Pacheco-Esquivel J, Carrasco-Rueda F, *et al.* (2014) Zombie bugs? The fungus Purpureocillium cf. lilacinum may manipulate the behavior of its host bug Edessa rufomarginata. *Mycologia* **106(6):** 1065–72. doi: 10.3852/13-264.

Enright MC, Robinson DA, Randle G, *et al.* (2002) The evolutionary history of methicillin-resistant Staphylococcus aureus (MRSA). *Proc Natl Acad Sci USA* **99(11):** 7687–92.

Hirsch EB, Raux BR, Lancaster JW, *et al.* (2014) Surface microbiology of the iPad tablet computer and the potential to serve as a fomite in both inpatient practice settings as well as outside of the hospital environment. PLOS One. 9(10): e111250. Doi: 10.1371/journal.pone.0111250. eCollection 2014.

Horie M, Honda T, Suzuki Y, *et al.* (2010). Endogenous non-retroviral RNA virus elements in mammalian genomes. *Nature* **463(7277):** 84–7. doi: 10.1038/nature08695.

Horie M, Kobayashi Y, Suzuki Y, *et al.* (2013) Comprehensive analysis of endogenous bornavirus-like elements in eukaryote genomes. *Philos T R Soc B* **368(1626):** 20120499. doi: 10.1098/rstb.2012.0499.

Kilmarx PH, Clarke KR, Dietz PM, *et al.* (2014) Ebola virus disease in health care workers — Sierra Leone. *Morb Mortal Wkly Rep* **63(49):** 1168–71.

Leroy EM, Baize S, Volchkov VE, *et al.* (2000) Human asymptomatic Ebola infection and strong inflammatory response. *Lancet* **355(9222):** 2210–5.

Matanock A, Arwady MA, Ayscue P, *et al.* (2014) Ebola virus disease cases among health care workers not working in Ebola treatment units — Liberia, June-August, 2014. *Morb Mortal Wkly Rep* **63(46):** 1077–81.

Miranda HC, Nunes SO, Calvo ES, *et al.* (2006) Detection of Borna disease virus p24 RNA in peripheral blood cells from Brazilian mood and psychotic disorder patients. *J Affect Disord* **90(1)**: 43–7. doi:10.1016/j.jad.2005.10.008

Mongkolsamrit, S, Kobmoo, N, Tasanathai, K, *et al.* (2012) Life cycle, host range and temporal variation of Ophiocordyceps unilateralis/ Hirsutella formicarum on Formicine ants. *J Invertebr Pathol* **111** (3): 217. doi:10.1016/j.jip.2012.08.007

Piercy TJ, Smither SJ, Steward JA, *et al.* (2010) The survival of filoviruses in liquids, on solid substrates and in a dynamic aerosol. *J Appl Microbiol* **9**: 1531–9.

Rao S, Scattolini de Gier N, Caram LB, *et al.* (2009) Adherence to self-quarantine recommendations during an outbreak of norovirus infection. *Infect Cont Hosp Epidemiol* **30(9)**: 896–9. doi: 10.1086/598346

Sagripanti JL, Rom AM, Holland LE. (2010) Persistence in darkness of virulent alphaviruses, Ebola virus, and Lassa virus deposited on solid surfaces. *Arch Virol* **155(12)**: 2035–9. doi: 10.1007/s00705-010-0791-0.

Shaib *et al.* (2014) Ebola Virus Disease Outbreak — Nigeria, July–September 2014. *Morbidity and Mortality Weekly Report.*

Wells WF. (1934) On air-borne infection: study II. Droplets and droplet nuclei. *Am J Hyg* **20**: 611–18.

Wilder-Smith A, Teleman MD, Heng BH, *et al.* (2005) Asymptomatic SARS coronavirus infection among healthcare workers, Singapore. *Emerg Infect Dis* **11(7)**: 1142–45.

Wichmann D, Schmiedel S, Kluge S. (2014) Isolation in patients with Ebola virus disease. *Intensive Care Med*, Dec 11, 2014. [http://link.springer.com/article/10.1007%2Fs00134-014-3582-3].

Yolken RH, Jones-Brando L, Dunigan DD (2014) Chlorovirus ATCV-1 is part of the human oropharyngeal virome and is associated with changes in cognitive functions in humans and mice. *Proc Natl Acad Sci USA* **111(45)**: 16106–11. doi: 10.1073/pnas.1418895111.

5

"How Cruel is That?"

As the Ebola crisis began to grip the consciousness of the western world, concerns of research on viruses initiating a pandemic of flu much worse than Ebola guinea were mounted by a group of scientists called The Cambridge Working Group in July 2014. In August 2014, Dr. Marc Lipsitch of the Harvard School of Public Health pushed for a meeting on the issue in an Op-ed article in *The New York Times* (Lipsitch, 2014). In October 2014, the White House suspended government-funded research that could lead to a gain of function in three infectious agents: Influenza, SARS and MERS. Gain-of-function studies are usually animal studies in which the virus' genome is modified specifically to cause the infectious agent to become more pathogenic, or to increase its transmissibility among mammals by respiratory droplets. The risk and value of such studies are being deliberated by the NIH, the National Science Advisory Board for Biosecurity (NSABB) and the National Research Council of the National Academies. Among the concerns cited were statistics on the loss and release of laboratory animals. In his article in *The New York Times*, Marc wrote:

> *Between 2003 and 2009, there were 395 "potential release events" and 66 "potential loss events" in American labs involving select agents, a category that includes many of the most lethal bacteria and viruses...*

The proposed value of such studies is to allow researchers to stay one step ahead of the viruses: To discover ways in which an already dangerous, contagious pathogen may become more pathogenic, or more virulent, and thus be one step closer to developing a vaccine should nature replicate their efforts in the lab.

The Cambridge Working Group is really a movement, playing the role of a conscious: Once again, has our technological ability to do something in science surpassed society's ability to deal with the ethical and moral questions?

"How Cruel is That?"

Such a movement, says Ken Kam, president and CEO of Marketocracy, is needed to shake up the FDA's insistence on the use of randomized placebo-controlled clinical trials for new drugs for EVD and other diseases. Ken and I chatted after I read his article in *Forbes Magazine* ("If You Had Ebola, Would You Want a Placebo," December 2014) in which he asked very poignant, probing and appropriate questions on the ethics of current clinical research:

> *(The FDA wants) patients to enroll in a clinical trial for the unapproved drug and take a risk that they will be randomly selected for the placebo group, which means they will get nothing more than "supportive care." How cruel is that? You take patients who are literally at death's door, give them the hope of getting access to a promising drug, but then end up giving maybe half of them a placebo.*
>
> *Why do we have to subject new Ebola patients to the risk that they will only get supportive care? Aren't there already enough Ebola patients who received only supportive care to serve as the placebo group? If there isn't enough data from the 9,000 or so people who have already contracted Ebola in the past year for the CDC and FDA to quantify the impact of various types of supportive care, then spend the money to develop the data from the continuing stream of patients who are currently receiving nothing more than supportive care.*

Ken is correct in his concerns here; someday, cultural anthropologists could comment on how cultural and behavioral changes are needed to improve the FDA's flexibility with respect to study design, so that eased restrictions can allow each study to help stem the spread of the disease. Dogmatic practices on study design like traditional burial practices in Western African peoples, can hamper efforts to stop the spread of disease.

For many, the FDA is being irresponsible: They are ignoring the hard-won gains in knowledge made by people who have published new approaches to study design, and on the benefits over pure random allocation. In their institutionalized behaviors and the position that only one type of clinical trial will be accepted, which seem overly starched, they act as if there is no risk of pandemic.

The FDA has published a position article in favor of randomized clinical trials of new EVD treatment going forward without upgrading the baseline of care to best available practice (Cox *et al.*, 2014). While the FDA has also said they might consider anecdotal evidence, there is actually little evidence of their use of such evidence in the past. In clinical trial design, complex does not mean biased. There are many, many robust and valid alternative trial designs that can lead to unbiased results. Other types of study aims seem especially warranted for EVD. These include Treatment X vs. Treatment Y with a common control (Koss and Goodman, 2014), and dose effects (where everyone on the trial gets some drug, and there is no placebo).

That way everyone has a shot at improving. Also, confounding is a complex issue, and on this issue, the FDA has made a mistake with regard to requiring best support care, too. The "best supportive care" in Africa under a trial that will render data acceptable to the FDA will include proper hydration. Higher standards of care are available and are in use on EVD patients in the US and Europe, including ventilators, and dialysis. Higher standards of care are available and are in use on EVD patients in the US and Europe, including ventilators, and dialysis. Even medical thermometers are scarce in many parts of West Africa. One study (WHO Ebola Response Team, 2014) actually recorded "febrile" and "not febrile" in a qualitative manner:

> *Fever was defined as a body temperature above 38°C; however, in practice, health care workers at the district level often do not have a*

medical thermometer and simply ask whether the person's body tem-
perature is more elevated than usual.

If the best care includes these best available care requirements, they amount to is too much of a variable in trial, and the trial will, as result of those changes, tend to be uninformative on the treatment effect for most African patients. This type of care will be largely irrel-evant to the vast majority of people in Africa who will die of EVD in the foreseeable future. They will not receive anything near the "best supportive care"; most won't even make it to an Ebola treatment center even if a drug becomes widely available, so a trial that updates the care to the standards required will be made (scientifically) entirely irrelevant to the majority of EVD patients in Africa.

This fact is reflected upon by Dr. Lewis Rubinson, who recounted (Rubinson, 2014) his deeply personal thoughts while contemplating the outcome after pricking his thumb with a nee-dle while working in an Ebola Treatment Unit at the Kenema Government Hospital (KGH) in Kenema, Sierra Leone:

> *I now just had to wait for the future to find out what would be the consequence of the needle stick. It was also very hard for me to recon-cile that I was not ill and likely never to be ill, but I was to be assisted with tremendous resources to get me back home. I am extremely grate-ful for all of those who made that happen. At the same time, many West Africans were actually ill or dying with EVD, and most were unable to get anything beyond very basic healthcare. This truth would continue to plague me throughout my experience… (were) the aero-medical evacuation, PEP, and overall resource expenditure overkill for the risk? I remain ambivalent. The risk was real, but it was far from a foregone conclusion that I would develop EVD. If the health-care infrastructure was more functional in Sierra Leone, I could have undergone evaluation and possible PEP in that country. I am glad that tremendous resources are available for persons who may contract EVD. I just wish that that they were available to all and not just the handful of expatriate responders.*

Egregious, irresponsible, random experimentation should always be eschewed. In Lakka, Sierra Leone, 14 health care workers walked out over what they saw as overly aggressive experimental use of a heart drug, amiodarone, for the treatment of *Ebolavirus*. They walked out because it was being administered in a haphazard manner without heart monitors, in some cases without consent, and the health care workers feared the treatment could be harming patients. In some cases, the application of the drug took precedence over baseline care. Amiodarone was not one of the 53 drugs that made the GP1GP2 inhibitor screen by Dr. Adolfo Garcia-Sastre.

This is also not the type of "science" this epidemic needs.

In a valid experiment, you change one thing at a time. To upgrade the baseline of care throughout Western Africa is ethical, of course, and a laudable goal. That alone may prove to help more than drugs. But it is not practicable. To evaluate a new treatment and change the clinical standard at the same time could jeopardize the relevance of the treatment effect for the general population. The FDA wants to change the baseline from historical for all placebo controlled trials, and then say that the historical data are irrelevant. That's not a good move; it may delay trials. What works locally might not work globally, but what is needed locally might be sufficient. How will we know if the treatment might only work at all under a best-care scenario, and not in the situation where there is no running water, or electricity?

In addition to testing in the actual, relevant clinical conditions, i.e., status quo, trials should also be run in new clinical settings, to ensure the drug's effectiveness for western medical settings. Right now the relevant clinical population does not have best care available, so let trials run with, and without it. The FDA, like so many other institutions involved in this crisis, is not using all of the tools that they have. As a result, they are not letting society benefit from knowledge gained more rapidly via alternative strategies to clinical studies.

The FDA does not approve drugs or devices themselves for compassionate use; instead, they approve specific uses of a drug or device. According to the US News and World Report, they approve nearly 1,000 specific uses for specific patients per year. While there is no list of drugs or treatments approved for compassionate use, a search of clinicaltrials.gov for open trials reveals that out of the 17,956 current open trials for treatments and drugs, only 381 qualify for accrual of patients for "Expanded Access" or "Compassionate Use." There is no official list of drugs or treatments that are currently approved for compassionate use, as the FDA considers each request for compassionate use on a case-by-case basis, so ostensibly the FDA should be able to produce thousands of instances of compassionate use. It would seem that due diligence means that the FDA would report the percentage of patients who benefit from compassionate use, but those numbers are not available.

There are currently eight different drugs at various stages of development (*New York Times*, Oct 23, 2014). Two drugs (Zmapp™ and VSV-EBOV) have passed only animal trials; all eight have been tried in health volunteers. Michael Duncan was treated under a fast-track mechanism with Brincidofovir, but he did not receive any transfusion from survivors due to blood type mismatch. Only two have been tested using small and large groups of patients (Brincidofovir and Favipiravir). The FDA has granted expanded access to some of these drugs. Dr. Anthony Fauci testified in the US House Oversight Hearings that the plan, at the time, was to secure proper information on dose and safety for these treatments, then any that qualify would be taken into "expanded trials," where larger numbers of individuals could be treated. He indicated that the first trials would include health care workers at the front lines of the Ebola epidemic.

Trials being conducted by Doctors Without Borders (MSF) are not placebo-controlled. On December 26, they released a statement, including the appropriately non-confounded study design for the drug favipiravir in Guinea:

> *All new patients arriving at the MSF Ebola Treatment Centre in Guéckédou are informed about the possibility of receiving the experimental treatment and can elect to participate in the study or not. Those who do not wish to be given the new treatment will receive the same supportive care as those who do, but without the administration of trial drug.*

(MSF, Dec 26, 2014)

Dr. Michael Osterholm, in his presentation at Johns Hopkins University, likened the challenge of public health and the medical community in Western Africa fighting Ebola to that of neurosurgeons being put to the task of brain surgery armed only with a sledgehammer and an axe. He cited how Doctors Without Borders has been criticized for proceeding in trying to treat EVD in some places without IV treatment, and lauded them for doing the best they can given the circumstances. This is far cry from best available care, and yet, scientifically, a superior study design given the clinical realities.

That said, now that western medicine is coming to Western Africa, if databases could be constructed tracking patients under specific regimes of care, matched sampling procedures could make the use of historical data even more relevant as a control. This could bring down the cost of clinical trials for diseases beyond EVD. With more than 16,000 cases of Ebola in Africa, we could surely find a few hundred past cases selected to match the clinical care regime of those on the trial. This speaks to the desperate need for a unified approach to medical record keeping in Ebola treatment centers in every country. This will prove most difficult when even the record keeping devices themselves cannot be decontaminated.

On a larger scale, within the context of clinical trials, the FDA also knows about the alternatives to completely randomized placebo-controlled trials; some of these other designs are more powerful than complete randomization, and are also relatively compassionate compared to placebo trials. Let's call them, generally, "Alternatively Randomized Clinical Trials," or ARCTs. These include response-adaptive designs, match/mismatch designs, and many, many other designs.

In response-adaptive designs, patients on a placebo arm would be monitored for signs of immunoresponse to the virus. Those who failed to produce large quantities of antibodies, or who appear to be rapidly declining, would be moved from the placebo arm to the treatment arm. Data from patients dropping from trials is handled by statisticians via methods called "censoring." In the case of EVD, we know that patients who mount a significant immune response tend to survive. Their viremia tends to decline in the second week of the disease. Those who fail to mount a response die. In more detail, there are two types of immune responses, leading to anti-Ebola antibodies and T-cells, and those who mount both have a better outcome (Baize *et al.*, 1999; Kash *et al.*, 2006; Wauquier *et al.*, 2010). During the course of clinical trial, patients with poor immunologic indicators could be switched to the treatment arm.

The FDA has had a "Draft Guidance" on the web since 2010 titled "Guidance for Industry Adaptive Design Clinical Trials for Drugs and Biologics." This 50-page document carries the disclaimers:

**This guidance document is being distributed
for comment purposes only**

and

Contains Nonbinding Recommendations
Draft — Not for Implementation

and

FDA's guidance documents, including this guidance, do not establish legally enforceable responsibilities. Instead, guidances describe the Agency's current thinking on a topic and should be viewed only as recommendations, unless specific regulatory or statutory requirements are cited. The use of the word should in Agency guidances means that something is suggested or recommended, but not required.

The guidance has been available for four years "for comment." For many in biomedical research, this is no way to govern. This "passive aggressive" approach is deplored by many involved in biomedical and clinical research. Again, we can see, the focus is on accountability, and it is not an enabling process. Given this document, the FDA has not officially come down on the topic one way or the other; thus, they cannot be criticized or held accountable for the effects of their stalwart position on RCTs. But you're wasting your time if you don't heed the implied official guidance.

If you read the entire document, it would leave you with the impression that the FDA's approach appears to be "prove it to me," as opposed to "this is how these studies could be done." In reality, this document exists as a more or less definitive communication to the clinical trials community's oft-repeated request for approval of treatments with safety and efficacy demonstrated in studies that, for practical reasons, use randomization approaches other than "complete" randomization. A close read reveals a litany of *possible* pitfalls of such studies, without any assessment of how likely those pitfalls may be, and at times no or at most insufficient information on the alternative methods and steps that can be used to avoid such pitfalls. We need a research-enabling position on this area from the FDA, and we needed it 10 years ago.

With all of the types of study designs mentioned in the guidance, the FDA, for the most part, falls back on a single type: (Completely) randomized clinical trials. The FDA was more direct in their position article in the *NEJM* (Cox *et al.*, 2014). In the *NEJM* Perspective article, they state that RCTs are preferred in part because historical controls (outcomes for the thousands who have died) may not reflect the outcome if they were given best available supportive care (BASC). People on clinical trials, it is thought, should be given proper basic care, and this has clearly not been the case for tens of thousands of patients in Africa. They argue that the only context in which a significant effect of an experimental treatment can be properly interpreted is BASC treatment vs. BASC placebo. However, it is altogether too clear that any field use of any experimental drug would have to be rolled out into a setting where the BASC was not that of the clinical trial, but was more similar to that of the historical data.

In their non-binding guidance, the FDA warns against spurious Type I errors that might be induced from other designs. However, they miss an important point: Other types of randomization also exist; they are more informed, and can yield higher power. Statistical power is the ability of a researcher to tell if there is difference in a measurement from two populations of interest when, in fact, there is a difference. Take, for example, bird wing length. An ecologist might wish to determine, objectively, whether the length of wing of a particular bird is different between high and low elevation populations. They would be expected to use a sample size of around 30 birds per group, take the average within each group, and use any of a number of statistical tests to determine if the average wing length differs. If it does, they are said to reject the null hypothesis that the lengths are the same. The larger the sample size for each of the two groups, the more precise the averages are, and the easier it is to be sure there is a difference when, in fact, there is. This attribute of a study is called statistical power, and it is given due consideration in every clinical trial. The usual tests to determine whether to reject the null hypothesis assume that the individuals are randomly sampled from the two populations.

For studies involving treatment with novel drugs, the two study populations, or cohorts, are created by a process called "allocation." When the FDA discusses "randomized clinical trials," the "random" part is the allocation: Patients are simply randomized to, say, the placebo or the treatment group. There are methods like covariate matching that can be used during random allocation of patients to treatment and placebo groups. Such methods can increase power by *reducing* unwanted spurious correlations of the main measurement of interest and other measurements that are not necessarily of direct interest to the study. Such spurious outcomes are guaranteed for some percentage of trials via complete randomization. When I used to teach a course in study design at the University of Pittsburgh, one of the most popular papers by far among my students was Aickin's paper "Beyond Randomization" (Aickin, 2002). Most people who read this paper, and the rest of Aickin's literature on the topic, come to the same conclusion: They provide unbalanced, high-powered study designs that are just as valid as purely randomized trials, with smaller sample sizes. Because they control so many variables simultaneously, such designs may, in fact, be superior to purely randomized trials. Aicken's papers should be required reading for every statistician employed and hired by the FDA.

For the most part, by rejecting data from studies that use ARCT designs, the FDA is saying ARCTs and others are too complex, and there are risks, so unless the study is completely randomized, the results will not be acceptable and the product will not be approved because otherwise they may be held accountable for a bad study that might leak through. The document spends an excess amount of space in laying out the pitfalls and insufficient attention is paid to the benefits of adaptive and other designs. The FDA's *NEJM* position has the unfortunate effect of cutting the use of more creative, yet still objective and unbiased, designs off at the knees.

A mentor of mine, Dr. Sam Wieand, used to hint about his frustrations on these matters over the lack of progress in clinical work due to what he called "foot-dragging" by the FDA in the allowance of data from non-standard clinical trials. Over his lattes, and my coffee, we would discuss my ideas on computational matching algorithms, and together we would marvel over the possible improvements in ovarian cancer biomarker study designs. We would then lament the futility in considering such advances in research methodology due to the FDA's "foot-dragging," because it would invariably cause clinical researchers to be reluctant to try study designs other than those they knew the FDA would accept. We knew the other designs were equal to, or superior, to those required by the FDA. Sam certainly did his part, and tried to help popularize clever methods in study design that, in some ways, were superior to those seen by the FDA as "gold standards," especially for case/control biomarker development studies (Weiand and throughout, 2005). He was a gentleman, and a true objectivity. Sam was a stickler for honesty, and a highly ethical man. He once discovered scientific misconduct in a breast and bowel cancer study. The study involved thousands of patients; data had been falsified in three. Sam and others found the fraud by checking data against public death records. Nothing escaped Sam.

He was also, politically, more subtle than most. But he had a fierce belief that things could be better. His legacy lives on: Similar methods inspired by his ideas have recently been used with great success demonstrating quite robustly the high value of chemoresponse assay in ovarian cancer (Tian *et al.*, 2014):

We used a match/mismatch analysis assess whether cross-drug response and correlated assay results across different therapies limit the predictive ability of the assay. This simple approach, evaluating the ability of the assay to predict patient outcome based on the assay result for the clinically administered therapy (match) as compared with a randomly selected treatment assay result for the same patient (mismatch), showed that the association of outcome and assay result for match was stronger than for mismatch (HR: 0.67 vs 0.81, respectively), indicating that a patient receiving an assay-sensitive therapy would be more likely to experience a better outcome than a patient treated empirically.

This study shows that their assay works better than chance at choosing which chemotherapy treatments would provide the best outcomes for patients. Now, oncologists of course do not choose chemotherapy prescriptions by chance; they follow protocols. For various reasons, patients in most cancer types end up with roughly the same treatments. The ChemoFX™ assay, and other assays like it, can benefit the patient in two ways that oncologists sometimes miss. First, if the assay predicts the agents that they themselves were likely to pick anyway, the oncologist might see this information as superfluous, and redundant to what they know. That is not the patient's experience, however. For each treatment, the patient has to consent. When an oncologist chooses the same treatment that a chemoresponse assay has predicted will work, the patient has a boost in confidence in the outcome. They have something much more valuable than knowledge or certainty that a test will work: They have more reason to *hope*.

The second benefit is in the case of the potentially rarer outcome: The assay and the oncologist disagree. In these cases, the negative effects of using an ineffective, but still chemically potent, chemotherapeutic agent are two-fold: First, the patient need not suffer side effects from a treatment that may not have any positive effect on their outcome. Second, and most importantly, the patient does not waste precious time receiving ineffective treatments, and can spend that time trying to determine, with their doctor, hopefully informed by the chemoresponse assay, which treatment options they *should* pursue. The value of the information provided to these types of patients cannot be underestimated.

For Ken Kam, the Ebola example is, hopefully, going to provide a watershed moment for shining a bright light on what's wrong with clinical trials research in the US, and it may prove to do just that. His inspirations are similar to my own: We both have lost a parent to cancer. His father was dying of lung cancer; with all of the available clinical options exhausted, they could not complete the extensive paperwork in time for his father to enroll in any clinical trials. They also could not succeed in securing compassionate use allowances for unapproved drugs in time. Ken's personal experience is not his only source of frustration. Ken founded and ran Novoste Corporation, and successful developed and brought a novel cardiac catheter to market, so he knows firsthand something about grueling FDA regulatory processes. He got out of the business of running companies in part because of the highly bureaucratic processes involved. He was not optimistic about additional successes due to the sometimes oppressive restrictions on the research processes.

He's not alone. I was once contacted by FDA scientists interested in seeing my Clinical Decision Modeling System (CDMS; Lyons-Weiler and Shi, 2007) submitted to the FDA as a Voluntary Data Submission just so the statisticians there could see that there were different ways of thinking about clinical trials. CDMS allows one to model millions of possible combinations of clinical tests for diagnostics in different orders of use, considered sensitivity, specificity, and the cost of each test. I designed the method and Harry (Haiwen Shi) built the software for me because the aim of biomarker development studies being conducted at the time was to "one-up" existing methods of diagnosis, instead of studying the context of an existing clinical workflow, and were seen as potentially augmenting current clinical care when used in combination. The person contacting me from within the FDA expressed deep frustrations over the huge number of studies rejected by the FDA because the sample sizes of the study could not be made to produce "sufficient power" using standard power calculations. What the FDA statisticians ignore is the fact that if a study already has produced a significant result, the sample size has already proven empirically to be sufficiently large to allow the test to have sufficient power. This is well-known. They focus on the fear that a study result could be an artifact of high variance. This is odd, because large variances are well known for making results not significant; in statistics speak, they usually *reduce* the probability of making a wrong inference of a significant results (a Type I error).

I hate to put it so bluntly, but it's true. People are dying, and companies are going out of business because of the intransigence of the FDA on these formal issues. They hold all of the cards in science. Science is supposed to be conducted as an open society. The company that grew my sister's triple negative breast cancer and tested a panel of chemotherapy agents, successfully predicting which chemotherapy agents would be most effective for her tumor, has successful demonstrated the utility of their assay using match/mismatched design of analysis (Tian *et al.*, 2014).

Sometimes the study designs required by the FDA are seen as draconian; sometimes, they are impossible. In chemoresponse studies, one cannot expect any oncologist to willfully subject their patient to an arm in a study design in which their actual chemotherapy options are done without consultation to a test that determines whether the treatment will work or not. If the chemotherapy fails to kill the cancer cells in a test tube, what oncologist could ethically determine that the clinical course for that patient should not be altered for the sake of the study, especially if past correlation studies have shown very high concordance of the efficacy *in vitro* (in the test tube) and *in vivo* (in patients)? While their tests can prevent people from wasting time on ineffective treatment, and try other approaches that might show benefit, given the *NEJM* position paper, the FDA will simply not consider data from anything other than a completely randomized clinical trial.

If society is going to benefit from the advances made in treatments, including drugs, procedures, and devices, a real, meaningful and consistent shift in the FDA's position is desperately needed on these issues: (1) Allowing the use of data from non-canonical study designs in all types of trials (not just those mentioned here, and not just those for Ebola treatments), and (2) the approval of results with "proven power," which would radically improve the translational success of research in the US. In our discussion, Ken Kam and I both wondered whether companies that have experimental drugs in other countries not held back by seemingly outdated methodological strictures would surge ahead of those in the US with successful clinical trials. The regulatory quagmire and dogmatic adherence to such a small slice of the valid study design spectrum is costing the US jobs, returns on investments that lead to intellectual property, and our health.

Ken's mission is to put the public in the position of being in the shoes of a patient being asked to enroll in a trial with some of the patients condemned to die without hope of benefit from the study because the design includes a placebo control. Some drugs, at the wrong dose, can elicit negative side effects. An example of this is TKM-Ebola from the company Tekmira. This drug, for example, when used in high doses on humans, elicited a cytokine storm — the same symptom that occurs near the end stage of Ebola — potentially accelerating the disease progression. Dangerous side effects are a rationale for a slow-moving bureaucracy. However, it would seem that the company would have noted such side effects under a compassionate use. The focus should be on expediting existing progress — for which discovery of proper dose is an important step — not bringing the process to a halt (a "clinical hold"), which is what the FDA did when they suspended Tekmira's trial. The hold has now been lifted in light of the severity of the epidemic, and the dose finding adds important new knowledge with respect to the immunological battlefield.

I hope that Tekmira and other companies perform exquisite due diligence in each phase of their studies, and I also hope that the FDA will consider data from non-canonical study designs. Not just for EVD — other diseases kill many more people, and many, many putative diagnostics and treatments are held up by limited viewpoints. My mentor and friend Sam's mission was the same, but more generalized. His was the same mission of many doing *bona fide*, objective science: Producing demonstrably generalizable and reproducible results to reduce pain and suffering.

These progressive efforts should not be rejected and minimized by the FDA simply because the FDA is unwilling, or unable, to do the work necessary to consider the value of these other approaches to study design. And certainly no one should ever have to be asked to be condemned to die, or to have an increased risk of no benefit from chemo, or no benefit from a placebo, for such reasons.

Perhaps, during ESF8, there should be a process involving a rapid review of the need for observational compassionate use studies of novel treatments for outbreaks. Scientists are most comfortable with properly controlled studies, so cause and effect can be attributed to the proper factor. However, there are circumstances under which a knowledge claim is warranted even when one has a sample size of one, and no opportunity for a proper randomized controlled study with replicates. In 1974, policy makers in Canada had a difficult time believing that the chemical phosphorous, found in fertilizers and detergents, was responsible for algal blooms in lakes, to the point of suffocation of the microbial, other plant, and animal life (eutrophication). Canadian/American ecologist David Schindler and his colleagues performed a "double basin" lake experiment. They split one lake into two, by placing a vinyl curtain between two halves of a lake, and treated one half with carbon, nitrogen, and phosphorous, and the other half with just carbon and nitrogen. The resulting image (Schindler, 1974), is famous among ecologists. It shows a screen of green algae on the treated side of the lake, and clear water on the untreated side, and was found to be very convincing by policy makers who "did not fully understand the scientific arguments" (Schindler, 2006). This was a study in which one lake served as its own control during the course of the lake's season.

The analogy in EVD is clear: Can an individual patient not serve as their own control during the course of their disease? Anyone with worsening symptoms past Day 4 is a high risk of death. Can we develop immunological correlates of outcome? While the lake experiment is simultaneous, with two halves of the lake split in space, in EVD compassionate use studies, the patient serves as their own control, separated by time. They are dying one day, and, hopefully recovering the next. Under canonical strictures of experimental design, it seems impossible to assign a positive turn in the course of the disease to the experimental treatment unless there is a sufficiently matched control that receives no treatment. But to many, Dr. Brantly's nearly instantaneous rebound is nearly as convincing as the lake photo. Ebola observational studies would also have an advantage over the lake study: The epidemic is large, and is replicated in three countries. It would be hard to argue that outcomes associated with a treatment that is found to cause patients to snap back into consciousness, replicated across numerous ETUs, are due, by chance, to some other factor. In a large epidemic, the need for compassionate use is made clear; the news and the blogosphere are filled with stories that drive the point home. Plus, there not enough experimental drugs to go around, so there should be plenty of controls who do not receive any treatment contemporaneous to any particular treatment arm. To algae, the lake is an ecosystem. To *Ebolavirus*, our bodies are the same, and the patient's will, or desire to live, or belief they will survive have little to do with the outcome. To require placebo control in *Ebolavirus* studies would be the same as requiring Dr. Schindler to have poured mock phosphorous as a placebo because perhaps the will of the experimenter brought about the massive and complete algal bloom.

The FDA's position is one based on political risk management. Clinical trials must be considered for two factors: The effectiveness of the treatment (efficacy), and the well-being of the patients (safety). The risk of the FDA's oversight being seen as a contributing factor to deaths due to side effects of a drug that was given to patients is transparent. The risk of the FDA's oversight being identified as a factor in the deaths of patients on clinical trials who did not receive an effective treatment is cryptic. Similarly, the FDA has never been called to a hearing with Congress to answer to complaints about deaths due to drugs they did not approve. This topic is analyzed thoroughly in a must-read article (Coriera, 2014).

The FDA's risk management policy was laid bare by Ebola, especially due to the graphic nature of the deaths to be expected for people on placebo-controlled trials.

I read a story of doctors struggling with ethics of bothering to try to insert a needle in a little girl's arm for the fifth day in a row, knowing her body only accepted trivial amounts of hydration, knowing she would bleed from the site, knowing her blood vessels had weakened, while her spirit remained strong. They wondered if she would recover (*The Guardian*). Her name was Katiada. She lived in Port Loko, Sierra Leone. Her doctors, including Dr. Martin Deahl, are already balancing, for patients not enrolled in clinical trials, the needs for medical care, palliative care, and their own humanity. The disease is devastating families and entire villages. In the village of Joeblow, Liberia, east of Kakata, all of the mothers have been killed by EVD (Knapton, 2014). If these doctors could try something that *might* work, sanctioned by WHO, the FDA and the CDC, the observational studies themselves would eventually prove the medicine's worth, especially if the data were aggregated. The luxury of placebo-controlled trials does not exist in this setting.

Vaccine trials are another story altogether, and one which drug test trials could learn from. "Randomly vaccinating the population would be a poor design," my friend Jeffrey Townsend recently reminded me. Instead, the best design is a "ring trial," where the idea is to create a bubble of immunity around an outbreak by immunizing those at highest risk: Health care workers, people who bury the dead, and people who have been in contact with persons infected with *Ebolavirus*. I asked Jeffrey of his opinion on the FDA's call for placebo-controlled RCTs.

I think there is a larger question than whether a drug should be approved for use in the U.S.A. or not. This outbreak is not like anything we have ever dealt with. We are trying to stem this outbreak with using technologies in their nascent, rather than well-studied form, and this may require the use of some options that are not in the standard playbook.

On the issue of quarantining health care workers and others exposed to the virus, Jeffrey was equally eloquent:

Public officials are charged with a difficult task, to balance the public safety against individual liberties. While it's not my position to say whether any of those decisions have been right or wrong, it is clear that the CDC defaults to a null of hypothesis of supporting personal liberty.

My own thoughts are both less poetic and more sanguine: "Jeff, when the CDC and others came out and said: 'We know this disease, we are ready to handle an outbreak in the US,' are they not really are saying that they can handle it, unless it gets too large? In which case, they are logically saying: 'We are ready to handle it, unless we aren't,' which means they are really saying nothing at all." Jeffrey replied:

The US has been able to contain infectious spread as long as the number of cases is small. Our capacity would be much more strained if there were many, many in the US.

Most infectious disease experts in the US are not concerned that EVD could take hold as a dire threat in developed countries such as the US. When I asked Dr. Michael Osterholm what was the most important thing about Ebola he wished that the American public knew, his answer was two-fold:

They should know that this epidemic had — and still has — the potential to be utterly disastrous for much of Africa outside these three countries. The fact that it has not taken hold in more places is a result of a combination of good public health work, and luck. Second, they should know that likelihood of EVD taking hold in the US as it has in Sierra Leone, Guinea and Liberia is next to nil. We have shown that with the cases that we have had that we have the ability to contain and treat the disease.

Dr. Adolfo Garcia-Sastre is the director of the Global Health and Emerging Pathogens Institute with the Icahn School of Medicine at Mount Sinai in New York City. Adolfo, who led the team who screened over 4,000 FDA-approved compounds, predicts a lengthy period of time before clinical trials of any of these compounds for treating EVD. On the record, he told me that:

"The priority should be help people with treatments that are unlikely to be harmful, and very likely to be beneficial. There are already some drugs that are known to work in animal models, also known not to be toxic. Zmapp is one example. Antibodies are relatively safe, well characterized, and unlikely to do harm. I think they are our best chance to rescue people from dying. These should be a first priority. Once Ebola is controlled, then we could do the dose optimization studies of drugs. There are multiple that are likely to beneficial, if possible they should be used in combination. We should be focused on saving lives first, and, if we can, determining efficacy: we should piggy back getting some data."

The right to protect one's life is certainly a personal liberty, and many feel that no government agency should limit a person's right to fight against anyone or anything that threatens their life. In the US, "The Right to Try" movement (Leonard, 2014) is likened to "Stand Your Ground" laws which allow the use of deadly force against anyone threatening a person's life. Five states (AZ, CO, MO, LA and MI) have Right to Try laws that allow doctors, hospitals and manufacturers to bypass the FDA on compassionate use while immunizing them, and any supplier from any state, from prosecution. Even under FDA compassionate use protocols, patients are informed of the possibility of unknown adverse side effects. Plus, they can remove themselves from the experimental trial for any reason.

It's time for the CDC and the FDA to take Dr. Michael Osterholm's messages at his speech at Johns Hopkins University to heart:

One of the worst enemies we can have today is dogma. Dogma should be, at the first instance, the thing we jettison immediately ... do not fall into the trap of dogma. I see far too many today doing that for the fact that they want to reassure the public about A, B or C, and that is a dangerous path.

References

Aickin M. (2002) Beyond randomization. *J Altern Complem Med* **8(6):** 765–72.

Baize S, Leroy EM, Georges-Courbot MC, *et al.* (1995) Defective humoral responses and extensive intravascular apoptosis are associated with fatal outcome in Ebola virus-infected patients. *Nat Med* **5:** 423–6. doi: 10.1038/7422.

Corieri C. (2014) Everyone deserves the right to try: Empowering the terminally ill to take control of their treatment. Goldwater Institute, 2/11/2014. [http://www.goldwaterinstitute.org/article/everyone-deserves-right-try-empowering-terminally-ill-take-control-their-treatment]

Cox E, Borio L, Temple R. (2014) Evaluating Ebola therapies — the case for RCTs. *New Engl J Med*, Dec 3, 2014. 2350–1. doi: 10.1056/NEJMp1414145

Kash JC, Mühlberger E, Carter V, *et al.* (2006) Global suppression of the host antiviral response by Ebola- and Marburg-viruses: increased antagonism of the type I interferon response is associated with enhanced virulence. *J Virol* **80:** 3009–20. doi: 10.1128/JVI.80.6.3009-3020.2006.

Koss N, Goodman S. (2014) Trials Tempered by Compassion and Humility. *The New York Times*, Dec 1, 2014.

Knapton S. (2014) Ebola wipes out every mother in Liberian village. *The Telegraph*, Jan 5, 2015.

Leonard K. (2014) Seeking the Right to Try. *US News and World Report*, Nov 18, 2014.

Lipsitch M. (2014) Anthrax? That's Not the Real Worry. *The New York Times*, June 29, 2014.

MSF. (2014) Clinical trial for potential Ebola treatment started in MSF clinic in Guinea. [http://www.msf.org/article/clinical-trial-potential-ebola-treatment-started-msf-clinic-guinea]

Rubinson L. (2014) From clinician to suspect case: My experience after a needle stick in an Ebola treatment unit in Sierra Leone. *Am J Trop Med Hyg* pii: 14-0769. [http://www.ajtmh.org/content/early/2014/12/11/ajtmh.14-0769.long]

Schindler DW. (1974) Eutrophication and recovery in experimental lakes: implications for lake management. *Science* **184(4139):** 897–9.

Schindler DW. (2005) Recent advances in the understanding and management of eutrophication. *Limnol Oceanogr* **51:** 356–363.

Shi H, Lyons-Weiler J. (2007) Clinical decision modeling system. *BMC Med Inform Decis Mak* **7(1):** 23.

Tian C, Sargent DJ, Krivak TC, *et al.* (2014) Evaluation of a chemoresponse assay as a predictive marker in the treatment of recurrent ovarian cancer: further analysis of a prospective study. *Br J Cancer* **111(5):** 843–50. doi: 10.1038/bjc.2014.375.

Wauquier N, Becquart P, Padilla C, *et al.* (2010) Human fatal zaire Ebola virus infection is associated with an aberrant innate immunity and with massive lymphocyte apoptosis. *PLOS Negl Trop Dis* **4:** e837. doi: 10.1371/journal.pntd.0000837.

WHO Ebola Response Team. (2014) Ebola virus disease in West Aferica — the first 9 months of the epidemic and forward projections. *N Engl J Med* **371:** 1481–95.

Wieand HS. (2005) Chemotherapy sensitivity and response assays: are the ASCO guidelines for clinical trial design too restrictive? *J Clin Oncol* **23:** 3643–3644.

6

With Blinded Eyes

"We know how to control Ebola, even in this period," testified CDC Director Thomas Frieden.

"We also know fire," I quipped out loud, as I watched the testimony to the US House Oversight Committee. Ask most people how to fight fire, and they will first think: "Pour water on it." However, some fires, such as grease fires, are made much worse using water. The question is whether the observed genetic and protein variations in this strain from Guinea have changed the biological characteristics of the virus sufficiently such that certain details of the know-how and knowledge and perspective in the training of health care workers, or in the care of patients, has inadvertently made transmission more likely than it would have for *Zaire ebolavirus*. Herein lies the conundrum. Highly trained, advanced, and high-ranking officials in the UN, the WHO, the US and other countries with modern health care systems can easily see when citizens of African countries often appear to fail to see themselves in their own cultural context. Western medical experts are not as likely to see themselves as capable of falling into traps of practice, custom, and culture, or to appreciate the role that these practices may have, in some settings, in preventing improved understanding. They are drilled for knowing what they know, aiming high on exams in college to ensure entrance into medical school. They have all sought the sacred rite of healing people. The White Coat culture has its own staid traditions, and being a medical doctor commands a great deal of respect. Regardless of the perceived virtues of western medical practice, it would be a tragedy if we eventually find that a grave error has been made in treating this strain as if were the same as strains from past outbreaks. If this proves to be the case, it means that western medicine was outsmarted by a remarkably small percentage of nucleotide variation.

Dr. Frieden continued:

> *There will not be an outbreak here, barring a mutation... I would be very concerned if there were mutations in this virus. There are none.*

I closed my laptop and sat, stunned. I was examining the very mutations present in the sequenced genomes of Ebola from patients who died in 2014. The 2014 *Ebolavirus*.

How could he say this, I wondered, when the key report of the emergence of Ebola in the *New England Journal of Medicine*, the source of the data I was analyzing, published a few weeks earlier, clearly showed mutations accumulating? They had found distinct differences, and observed the frequencies of genetic variants changing over time in the transmission chains. Early patients had lower frequencies of some mutations, or more properly, polymorphisms, in the population of virus in their blood; later patients had higher frequencies. They had caught the virus evolving.

That day was the day I decided to enter into a relationship with *Ebolavirus*. Because I had left phylogenetics and molecular evolution to study cancer during my postdoctoral years, I often felt that there could be more to the story in molecular medicine than I was seeing in the case/control studies I worked on with colleagues. I found myself limited by preconceived notions that it was sufficient to study individual mutations on their own merit, and that for certain diseases in humans there were no gene–gene interactions (pleiotropy). Here was a problem not only worthy of my time, but a problem for which the most senior ranking official in the US Centers for Disease Control and Prevention left me with the impression that he was overlooking a great deal of the background of evolutionary processes. Perhaps, I thought, I could be found to be useful in this area.

This was not an easy undertaking for me; these events were happening just as my lay-off from the University of Pittsburgh was taking effect. I had spent 14 years helping medical researchers with their bioinformatics needs. For the last seven years, I was scientific director of the university's Bioinformatics Analysis Core. Budget cuts by Governor Tom Corbett and a low return on investment from the excellent algorithm development and data analysis services provided to the community in the form of federally funded grants led to closure of the Core. Unsure of what to do, I turned to a trusted mentor: My friend Bob Banerjee. Bob is one of the most contemplative, meditative and loving people I know. But he's his own type of guru: He and his colleague John McCann have sustained many spiritually and emotionally in the Pittsburgh region with their band "Corned Beef and Curry." Bob would try to tell you that it's the Jameson or the suds that provide the spirit, but if you ever get to see their show, you will see what I mean. Bob had heard about the lay-off and invited me to lunch. During our conversation, he gave me the encouragement I needed: He told me that the period of time serving others in my last position was the period of time for doing "that particular good." The question, Bob challenged me, was: *"What is the next particular good you're going to do?"*

Even being laid off, I had it easy compared to those suffering in Western Africa. As if fighting EBV in patients and stemming the spread of the disease weren't bad enough, Africans also must somehow determine if new cases are actually Ebola, or perhaps another, less lethal but still dangerous cousin, Lassa fever virus. Like Ebola, Lassa fever is a hemorrhagic disease. If Ebola takes hold in the US again, while our families and communities must make sure that flu-like symptoms are not actually due to *Ebolavirus*, doctors and patients in Western Africa must perform differential diagnosis between EV and Lassa fever. Moreover, during the 2014 outbreak, a second, independent outbreak emerged in the Democratic Republic of the Congo. That outbreak has apparently now ended; however, the thought that in a given year, we may be fighting two, or more strains, concerns me.

So I decided to go for a drive. It was a clear fall day, and I drove the hilly countryside around Pittsburgh. "What would be the most effective way to shut down this outbreak?" I pondered, still cooling off from the testimony debacle. Certainly we need to reduce transmission rates; that's why they isolate infected people. No, wait. They isolate people sick with Ebola, not infected, because they don't know who is infected. Maybe that's why it's so bad this time, I thought. What we needed, I realized, was a diagnostic sensitive enough to detect *ebolavirus* early, before symptoms. They were starting to screen people at airports, and I was rather sure that checking travelers from Western African countries for signs of fever would miss any who were not symptomatic. The questions focus on whether the person has been in contact with Ebola patients, attended funerals of Ebola patients, etc. The questions could be more effective — *Have you spent time with anyone sick with flu-like symptoms? Has anyone you spent time with recently died for any reason? Cause of death?* So the screening could help, but the questions would certainly miss some people who did not know they had been exposed. Just like we allow people to get sick with EVD, leading to transmission, cases would slip through. We need more sensitive screens, I thought, just like we need more sensitive tests. Perhaps, I thought, we should screen at the point of departure, and do a more thorough screen there, rather than do weak screens worldwide.

Then I had a flash of insight. Since we have been told that the disease cannot be transmitted prior to the onset of symptoms, the best way to shut down this outbreak (and prevent it from becoming an epidemic, which it was not yet, at the time) was to design a test capable of detecting Ebola *before* the immune system has a response. The priority was also emphasized in *Nature* magazine by David Heymann, one of the pioneers in the field (Heymann, 2014). He stressed early diagnosis and isolation of patients with fever as one of the key strategies learned from past outbreaks. I thought of the more technologically challenging problem: How could one detect *Ebolavirus* prior to any symptoms? I thought about the virus, the proteins on the coat. I thought about how the virus uses conformational changes in its proteins with ruthless efficiency. We could evolve a detector molecule of some kind, perhaps something like an artificial antibody. We could optimize its evolution using genetic algorithms to not only optimize the binding, but also, simultaneously, to have a large conformational state change capable of being detected. I envisioned a glass tube with a membrane inside, with part of the membrane sticking out the one open end. I envisioned an airport screener passing out these tubes, with each traveler removing a cap off the open end. I envisioned their saliva passively absorbed, and then the cap going back on, with the tube then being placed in a zip-lock type baggie. I then saw them looking at the tube, waiting for a color change. Positives to the left, negatives to the right. Thank you for flying with us, have a nice day. I had no idea how the test should or could be made, but I knew it had to rapid, reliable, safe and inexpensive.

Having been in bioinformatics for so long, I had plenty of time to become familiar with its cousin discipline, computational biology. Bioinformatics is primarily and at its core the study of DNA and protein sequences by people seeking ways to understand variation. Computational biology is more focused on the three-dimensional structures of RNA and amino acid sequences. I wondered if there were any computational biologists willing to work with me on my idea. What would it require?

I didn't really know who was working on genetic algorithm evolved protein structures for specific capabilities, but I knew of a place I could find out. I posted a query in the Computational Biology group on the social network, LinkedIn. I outlined the concept, and asked anyone who knew anyone who did this type of work in computational biology to please forward the message and have them contact me.

To create a novel means of detecting a virus means, at some point, you have to test the device with live virus. If political expediency led to the scientifically incorrect testimony of no mutations, to assuage the House Oversight Committee, as an answer to their politically motivated searing questions and commentary, then clearly there was a very messy, or some would say "delicate," situation, that

I had to deal with in approaching working with the CDC. Perhaps the director and his staff somehow missed the *NEJM* study? Perhaps they were so focused on every aspect of the fight against the disease that they missed the indications that this virus is different? However unlikely this scenario, it was a possibility. But then I thought about my sister's oncologist. Even if that oncologist had missed that report on low-dose tamoxifen, *he should have known*. The same seemed true to me with regard to Dr. Frieden's testimony. The testimony that appears to be designed to assuage the House Oversight, and the American public, was potentially spreading misinformation to medical personnel all across the US, and the world, as to what to expect of Ebola guinea.

It's natural for officials to want to report that they have the situation under control, and that they are prepared to handle whatever might come. But no one could miss the volume of linens and medical waste created by the treatment of Thomas Eric Duncan, and all the indications pointed to me that something was very different about this virus. The odds that Dr. Frieden did not know seem vanishingly small. What then, could explain the false, incorrect and (either way) misleading testimony to the House Oversight? I needed to know.

Through various organizations and communities, I am in contact with, and have collaborated with, hundreds of people. We help each other out with letters of support, letters of collaboration, by sharing data, and through other communications in support of grant writing efforts as a matter of routine. Such a request for a letter is rarely declined. I had contacted the CDC requesting a letter of commitment that if the first projects were successful, that we could count on them to conduct, with costs covered by funding from the consortium, tests of the device for early, pre-symptomatic utility with live virus in their BSL-4 laboratory. To my dismay, and surprise, my request for a letter for future support was declined, with a terse explanation that they already have assays that are being tested in the field. I thought that a simple letter, to agree to help us translate the device we hoped to build, would have been a very small favor to request; perhaps, again, they were too busy dealing with all of the other aspects of the Ebola crisis.

Two weeks later, a number of colleagues forwarded to me a letter of invitation to the scientific community from the White House to participate in a conference call. This call was to share the White House's agenda on Ebola for the immediate future. I was delighted. Here was a potential opportunity for me to set the record straight: To share with other scientists my concerns over the mutations that were, for all I knew, being ignored by the CDC and others working on Ebola diagnostics. The mutations could, in principle, hurt existing assays to detect *ebolavirus*, or the molecular signatures of *Ebolavirus*, because the molecular assays rely on the virus to provide information about its presence.

There are two main types of molecular diagnostic kits for Ebola and other RNA viruses. The first type checks a person's blood to determine if antibodies were produced by their immune system in response to the presence of a foreign protein, or antigen. This approach works after the immune system has detected the viral protein. Such assays work via the binding of antibodies on the assay that are specific to a protein found on the suspected infectious agent. The signal, or report, of the presence of the protein being tested for is reported by agents on the assay that light up when the protein is detected. This detection requires that the local protein sequence match that expected by the assay. Binding can fail, or be too weak to rise above the background. Given the need for these tests to be highly specific, the test can also, in principle, fail if the protein sequence within the targeted region has changed due to mutations.

The second type of assay is called RT-PCR, which stands for reverse transcription polymerase chain reaction. PCR has driven the last 30 years of research in molecular biology. In PCR, the actual DNA sequence, or in the case of RNA viruses, the reversely tran-scribed RNA, of the infectious agent is used as anchors for specific sites to which small stretches of matching, artificially produced DNA sequences, are bound (or annealed) at a specific temperature.

These small matching DNA sequences, or primers, have to be fairly specific, otherwise the reaction will not proceed. If a virus evolves away from the known template sequence at the sites corresponding to the primer annealing, a false negative, or "missed positive," could result. The result could be that a patient, soon to be sick with EVD, is sent home, or a health care worker given the all-clear to treat patients.

One of the frontliners, Dr. Robert Garry, professor of Microbiology and Immunology at Tulane's School of Medicine, was interviewed about his experiences in Sierra Leone. He was there doing research on Lassa fever with colleagues when EVD struck. He put it this way:

> *If the sequences of the virus are changing, then these PCR, what we call PCR primers, don't work as well or may not work at all. And that compromises our ability to get a good diagnosis for the virus and tell if the person actually has it or not. Unfortunately, there are cases popping up where the assays weren't sensitive enough and the person is not diagnosed until the person had gone away or it had affected other people. If you can't make a proper diagnosis of the infection, then there is a chance that the person will be turned back and they will infect other people and infect a health care worker, and we have cases of that, unfortunately, that continue to happen.*

> (Catalanello, 2014)

None of the existing assays work well in the early, presymptomatic phases of the disease. While testing suspected patients for EVD prior to any symptoms can, in principle, work, a negative result prior to symptoms, or prior to the 21-day "watchful waiting" period is meaningless. Only a positive result can be interpreted as definitive. Failure to understand this important aspect of diagnosis can have tragic consequences. Consider the case of Dr. Martin Salia (d. 2014) from Sierra Leone (d. 2014). Upon hearing that his test was negative for Ebola, his colleagues embraced him when he tested negative. Unfortunately, the test was negative *within the*

21 day watch period. The testing protocol failed this doctor, and his colleagues, because it was not sensitive enough, and was not able to detect the virus in an asymptomatic infected person.

The reasons for negative tests are likely varied, but they include that the person has to have sufficient viral load to cause an immunological reaction for the immunohistochemistry assays to work, or sufficient RNA from the virus in the blood for the RT-PCR reaction to work. These are late-stage conditions, at a time when the patient is also most likely capable of spreading the disease.

I also knew that if *Ebolavirus* changed rapidly over time via mutation, then any diagnostic assays would have to be developed anew for each outbreak. They would have to be tailored to the strain, like the vaccine for influenza. I had grave concerns given Dr. Frieden's testimony, that Ebola guinea had already evolved, or was evolving, away from the available molecular diagnostic assays, and that false negatives could result. False negatives could cause people to let down their guard, leading to transmissions.

Dialing into the White House conference call, I was hopeful to get an answer to the question of what types of assays are being tested in the field, and, more importantly, whether the known mutations shown to exist in the strain infecting patients to date in 2014 were taken into consideration for existing and new tests. The conference call was run as follows: All lines were muted, except at the end, where those who hit "*1" were called upon to ask a question. "*1" was like raising your hand.

The first message of the conference call was a reminder that this phone call was not for the press, rather, it was a plea to the scientific community to be responsible when speaking with the public about Ebola: Basically, to get our facts straight. The speakers emphasized the CDC party line that no one can catch Ebola from anyone unless they are symptomatic and have the virus.

Most faculty members doing research in the US are not capable of being politically outspoken because with each change of presidential administration and congressional majority party change, research funding priorities change. Sometimes, the changes are based on dogma. I interviewed a researcher in evolutionary biology who asked to not be identified. He recounted that, in the 1990s, upon taking the Senate and the House, conservatives in the US started exerting a good deal of influence on the funding agencies. After President Bush took office, the researcher had contacted a program officer at the National Science Foundation to inquire on the possible fit of the aims of research study to the funding priorities of a specific call for proposals. Dr. Rita Colwell was the Director of the NSF at the time, appointed by President George W. Bush. The program officer informed my source that the proposal was fine, but that they had been given — by word of mouth — the mandate that any proposal that included the term "evolution" was to be triaged, that is, returned unreviewed, to the proposal author (principle investigator). The proposal could be about evolution, but it could not include the term. To me, this is dogma ruling over science, and the practice should never be repeated.

There were a couple of additional speakers, and then the Q&A period. The first question came from an anthropologist, who wondered why the CDC and WHO did not call on sociologists and anthropologists so they could help communicate the truth about *Ebolavirus* to locals. We were informed by the questioner that cultures very greatly from region to region, and that a message useful in one region might not be as well received in other regions, and that the CDC and the WHO should consider working with the sociologists and anthropologists expert in each region for effective ways of integrating messages about Ebola to the local populations. "Great idea," I thought. I have subsequently learned that the Wellcome Trust Foundation has funded just this type of effort.

There was time for four questions. At the close of the third question, I hesitated. Should I hit "*1?" I wondered. "Oh, why not," I thought, "you only live once."

My two-question question was turfed to a member of CDC, the very person who turned down my request a week or so earlier for a letter of support for live-virus testing of a new type of assay. To my first question, he answered that they were working on all types of assays to detect *Ebolavirus*, for example, in hospitals, and airports. No details were provided on technicalities of specific tests.

I thought it odd, given that this call was for scientists. Scientists ask questions. He dodged that question. As for the mutations, we were told that yes, the impact of the mutations was being considered for the new tests. I was hoping to hear this, because I feared that the tests that were already in the field were designed and constructed before the mutations were reported in the *New England Journal of Medicine.*

After some closing statements by the host, that was the end of the call.

References

Catalanello R. (2014) Q&A with Tulane researcher on front line of Ebola outbreak. *The Times-Picayune*, Aug 28, 2014. [http://www.nola.com/health/index.ssf/2014/08/qa_with_tulane_researcher_who.html]

Heymann DL. (2014) Ebola: learn from the past. *Nature,* Oct 9, 2014.

7

Are We Asking the Right Questions and Solving All the Right Problem(s)?

You would have to search far and wide to find anyone involved in scientific and biomedical research that would say that a vaccine for Ebola should not be our first priority. At this point in the epidemic in Sierra Leone (early December), the news is not good, and worsening, and while a vaccine is important, at this point, it should not be seen as an exclusive priority. In Sierra Leone, schools and community centers that had been transformed into triage centers have been turned into make-shift full-time containment centers to isolate suspected cases of EVD (*NPR*, Morning Edition, Dec 5, 2014). The number of new cases per week in the first week of December had reached an all-time high for any country since the outbreak began: 537.

The differences between a containment center and an Ebola ward are stark. No one expects any of the patients in containment centers to survive. In Sierra Leone, these containment centers were originally designed for triaging patients to treatment centers. Because the treatment centers are full, the triage centers became *ad hoc* containment centers. Treatment in these places, if any, is palliative. The reason is a severe lack of resources. Health care workers do not have IVs, nor do they have the tests necessary to check electrolyte levels. And, like the rest of us, they have no way to reliably test whether a patient suspected of having EVD is infected prior to the end of the 21-day monitoring period. The international community has not pulled together the resources needed to fight the spread via effective treatment, and the disease is moving faster than the medical community. Much faster.

The concern has been that a vaccine might come too late (Kanapathipillai *et al.*, 2014; Cohen, 2014). Thousands of Sierra Leoneans will die unless IV bags, ventilators, clinical test kits and PPG are shipped from every country. More health care workers will contract the disease, severely curtailing the country's ability to contain its spread. Sierra Leone has about 0.3 doctors per 1,000 people. The US has 2.3. Expressed per capita, every death of a doctor Sierra Leone is like eight doctors dying at once in the US. As of November 23, 105 health care workers had died in Sierra Leone, making up a whopping 7.5% of the total deaths. If 800 health care workers died in the US from EVD, we would have an uproar, and an immediate change in policy. We must recognize this virus is different, yes. But we must also recognize that our view of the immediacy and urgency of the faults in our system looks different when we consider their impact on people abroad compared to their impact on ourselves.

While the epidemic in Africa is reason enough, a larger epidemic of Ebola in Western Africa also means EVD worldwide. In October 2014, a study by Bogoch and colleagues showed that an average of 2 to 8 passengers per month should be expected to depart Western Africa countries with Ebola (Bogoch *et al.*, 2014). They also noted that screening departing flights at three airports would be more efficient than screening incoming flights at a large number of destination airports. Cowling and Yu (2012) commented on the paper that many think it is wise to continue to monitor incoming flights from West Africa in part due to strained resources in the countries of origin.

Models such as those used in these studies are behind President Obama's statement that we can expect, with certainty, additional Ebola cases within the US. In September 2014, the worst-case scenario mathematical prediction by the CDC for the number of cases in West African countries was 1.4 million. If that number were ever reached, we were told, we could expect to see a few cases of Ebola in every major city in the US.

"We are Prepared to Handle an Ebola Outbreak in the United States"

This was among the forward-looking statements projected on major news outlets in the US. The bulk of the efforts of the CDC health care workers is to perform case finding and contact tracing, to identify people who should be isolated and watched, and to treat the sick. This is a complex, lengthy, and easily broken process. In the case of Patrick Sawyer, the outbreak in Nigeria was contained over the course of three months. That effort involved contact tracing that required 18,500 face-to-face interviews with 894 contacts, and resulted in the eventual diagnosis of EVD in 20 people (Shuaib *et al.*, 2014). Jim Yong Kim, President of the World Bank Group, reported the cost:

> *For Senegal, the cost to treat one patient and track all of his contacts was more than $1 million. For Nigeria, one infected person led to 19 other cases, and more than 19,000 contacts traced by over 800 health care workers at a cost of more than $13 million. In Guinea, Liberia and Sierra Leone, there are not one or 10 active transmission lines, but hundreds. Defeating Ebola now will cost billions — but it will spare the rest of the world from the spread of the virus, save lives in the countries, save money over the long term, and help the countries rebuild their economies.*

> — "The Path to Zero Ebola Cases." *NYT* op-ed,
> Jim Yong Kim, Dec 11, 2014

At the peak of the epidemic, tracing transmission lineages became futile: Those trying to do the work lost track. In October 2014, thousands of people in Sierra Leone were leaving their homes in search of food because the world had not responded earlier with sufficient aid. Modelers projected that if 70% of people infected with *Ebolavirus* in West African countries are isolated, the outbreak can be held constant. Disturbingly, they predict this benchmark would produce a steady-state outcome, not necessarily shutting the outbreak down. Even at numbers very close to zero, large resurgences could occur. When we consider that time is a major factor that determines the number of new mutations that will occur in a population, a steady-state of Ebola cases in Africa, or anywhere, is not a tenable outcome.

The ultimate value of vaccines to individuals is that they don't get sick. The ultimate value of vaccines is that they break the transmission chain. Prevention of transmission is certainly an important agenda item; including and beyond isolation of infected individuals, there are information campaigns designed to encourage people to not touch dead bodies, to stay away from fruit bats, and the like.

However, prevention of transmission could also be achieved via a radical shift towards improved, and earlier, diagnosis. Patients could be treated before they become symptomatic. A definitive early test is needed (recall the tragic consequences of Dr. Martin Salia's unfortunate and tragic false negative test). The world should take note that a result from available tests for Ebola prior to 21 (CDC) or 42 (WHO) days from suspected exposure is only meaningful if the results are positive: A negative test means little.

Remember the CDC's and the NIAID's official guidances state that one can only contract Ebola through:

> *Direct contact (through broken skin or mucous membranes in, for example, the eyes, nose, or mouth) with blood or body fluids (including but not limited to urine, saliva, sweat, feces, vomit, breast milk, and semen) of a person who is sick with Ebola.*

"Sick with Ebola" means "symptomatic." They believe that people who are not symptomatic do not shed the virus. Assuming this is true, then it would follow that detection of the virus prior to the presentation of symptoms would be an urgent priority: Patients diagnosed with EVD early seem to respond better to treatment, and the risk of incidental exposure of health care workers would be much lower if patients began treatment before the disease could manifest itself.

Early Diagnosis to Protect the Public Health

A diagnostic capable of detecting *Ebolavirus* in saliva prior to symptoms would be even better: It could allow treatment prior to symptoms, preventing symptoms and reducing contagiousness.

I am advocating, as a priority second only to vaccine, for the development of a new class of biosensor diagnostic for Ebola capable of detecting the virus in the saliva of asymptomatic individuals as the primary mechanism that will serve to shut down this, and any other, outbreak. Total population screening with tests capable of detecting even a minute amount of virus in saliva would allow the immediate triage of the ostensibly still "safe to treat" asymptomatic infected individuals. Treatment would prove more effective, and for each patient, less human suffering would have to be endured. In this disease, false negatives are vastly more costly than false positives.

The use of early diagnostics to allow early treatment, thus preventing possible transmissions, is clearly a public health measure, which fits an ethical priority (Dawson, 2015), by providing a highly effective means of mitigating the spread. There is one problem. No such diagnostic yet exists. The WHO has identified 18 candidate assays for the diagnosis of Ebola. None are reported to be capable of detecting the virus in asymptomatic persons. Drawing blood is risky. Saliva-based tests might be the safest; however, one lateral flow immunological assay mentions saliva, and the statistics from the one field tested shows that it suffers from low sensitivity (WHO Report).

Some reasonable priorities should be given due consideration:

1. Develop a diagnostic assay capable of detecting *Ebolavirus* in saliva in asymptomatic, including presymptomatic persons infected with *Ebolavirus*. This really is a most pressing priority:

If people with *Ebolavirus* infections can be isolated and treatment can begin before they have symptoms, the risk of transmission and spread will be made astronomically smaller.

2. Start treating people at high risk of *Ebolavirus* infection with plasma donations from convalescent patients (Gupta *et al.*, 2001; Lu *et al.*, 2014). Dose escalation experiments of convalescent serum therapy trials (passive immunotherapy) should be fast-tracked and they should be allowed to involve any number of people and various clinical settings. Although one study (Jahrling *et al.*, 2007) showed no effect of passive immunotherapy in rhesus monkeys, the most compelling evidence of clinical efficacy of this type of was the passive immunotherapy with convalescent-phase human blood used on 10 patients during the EVD outbreak in Kikwit in 1995; nine survived (compared to then historical baseline of 20% survivorship) (Mupapa *et al.*, 1999). In a follow-up study, antibodies from the survivors were shown to neutralize *Ebolavirus* (Rowe, 1999). At relatively low cost, large amounts of protective immunoglobulins could be produced (Maruyama *et al.*, 1999). The fact that the animal trial failed speaks to the growing concern that sometimes the outcomes of animal studies fail to predict the efficacy of treatments in human trials for other treatments and drugs. Some highly effective and important treatments in humans may be missed; such treatments work in mice, but not rhesus monkeys.

3. In the future, stores of immunoglobulins should be produced by WHO and CDC in anticipation of outbreaks (Lachmann, 2014).

4. Allow compelling results from treatment vs. treatment and dose vs. dose studies in addition to any "gold-standard" RCTs.

5. Recognize other unbiased study designs as valid, and allow compelling results from alternatively randomized clinical trials (ARCTs) with unbiased study designs, whenever possible.

6. Simplify compassionate use procedures for existing and novel treatments for Ebola. The FDA could invite Ebola Treatment Case Study Reports for both positive, and, importantly, negative outcomes. They could issue a standard form for data collection that could be online, emailed, faxed, or mailed. The data could

be compiled into one database, publicly available, ready for analysis by anyone willing to conduct their own analysis. I have created a draft form (Appendix 2).

7. Apple or Microsoft could build and donate clonable "instant IT infrastructure" into all Ebola treatment centers worldwide to gather clinical treatment and outcomes data. Create BSL4-level sleeves for tablets and cellphones that can be disinfected.

8. As is already underway, create "CDCs" in each of the countries where outbreaks are likely to take place; allow them to determine the suitability of the trials in their own countries, for their own clinical populations, so as to extract the most relevant information for the afflicted populations. What works locally might not work globally, but what is needed locally might be sufficient.

9. Pre-medical biology students should be required to have courses in evolutionary biology, molecular evolution, population genetics and study design so they can properly consider the sources of variation (mutation, migration) and the factors that remove or fix variation. These include random changes in frequencies due to small population size, a.k.a. drift, and changes in frequencies due to their effects on survival and reproduction, a.k.a. selection.

10. To prevent future outbreaks, start a campaign to vaccinate the people, and the wildlife (suspected of being reservoir hosts) in Ebola regions. Gorillas are woefully afflicted with Ebola outbreaks from time to time; for their own sake, too, perhaps we could tattoo gorillas given passive immunotherapy for all strains of *Ebolavirus* and those given saline and then see if, during the outbreak, those treated had better survival during the next outbreak.

11. Health care facilities should be prepared for massive volumes of waste, and sudden, perhaps increasingly projectile, vomiting.

References

Bogoch II, *et al.* (2014) Assessment of the potential for international dissemination of Ebola virus via commercial air travel during the 2014 west African outbreak. *The Lancet.* pii: S0140-6736(14)61828-6. doi: 10.1016/S0140-6736(14)61828-6.

Cohen J. (2014) Infectious disease. Ebola vaccine: little and late. *Science* **345**: 1441–1442.

Cowling B and H Yu H. (2014) Ebola: Worldwide dissemination risk and response priorities. *The Lancet* 2014. pii: S0140-6736(14)61895-X. doi: 10.1016/S0140-6736(14)61895-X.

Dawson AJ. (2015) Ebola: what it tells us about medical ethics. *J Med Ethics* **41(1)**: 107–10. doi: 10.1136/medethics-2014-102304.

Gupta M, Mahanty S, Bray M, *et al.* (2001) Passive transfer of antibodies protects immunocompetent and imunodeficient mice against lethal Ebola virus infection without complete inhibition of viral replication. *J Virol* **75(10)**: 4649–54.

Jahrling PB, Geisbert JB, Swearengen JR, *et al.* (2007) Ebola hemorrhagic fever: evaluation of passive immunotherapy in nonhuman primates. *J Infect Dis* **196 (Suppl 2)**: S400–3.

Kanapathipillai R, Restrepo AM, Fast P, *et al.* (2014) Ebola vaccine — an urgent international priority. *N Engl J Med.* doi: 10.1056/NEJMp1412166.

Lachmann PJ. (2014) Traditional passive immune therapy for emerging Ebola infection. *Emerg Microbes Infect* **3**: e81. doi:10.1038/emi.2014.87 [http://www.nature.com/emi/journal/v3/n11/full/emi201487a.html]

Lu S. (2014) Using convalescent whole blood or plasma as passive immune therapy for the global war against Ebola. *Emerg Microbes Infect* **3**:e80. doi:10.1038/emi.2014.86 [http://www.nature.com/emi/journal/v3/n11/full/emi201486a.html]

Maruyama T, Rodriguez LL, Jahrling PB, *et al.* (1999) Ebola virus can be effectively neutralized by antibody produced in natural human infection. *J Virol* **73(7)**: 6024–30.

Mupapa K, Massamba M, Kibadi K. (1999) Treatment of Ebola hemorrhagic fever with blood transfusions from convalescent patients. International Scientific and Technical Committee. *J Infect Dis* **179(1)**: S18–23.

NPR. (2014) World's Slow Response to Ebola Leaves Sierra Leone Villages Scrambling. *NPR Morning Edition*, Dec 5, 2014.

Rowe A. *et al.* (1999) Clinical, virologic, and immunologic follow-up of convalescent Ebola hemorrhagic fever patients and their household contacts, Kikwit, Democratic Republic of the Congo. *J Infect Dis* **179(1):** S28–35.

Shuaib F, *et al.* (2014) Ebola Virus Disease Outbreak — Nigeria, July–September 2014. *Morb Mortal Wkly Rep* **63(39):** 867–72. [http://www.cdc.gov/mmwr/preview/mmwrhtml/mm6339a5.htm]

8

Evolution is Real: Deadly Consequences of Dogma

In the months building up to international awareness of the seriousness of the outbreak, information campaigns were launched to inform locals of the terrible truth of EVD. Governments used pamphlets and signs and t-shirts labeled with three words as they sought to reassure people that Ebola is not a curse placed upon, or by a family member; that it is not a disease being given (on purpose) to locals by foreign medical staff; that, in fact, Ebola is Real.

My own reaction to Dr. Frieden's testimony was due not only to my deep and abiding academic interest in evolution and evolutionary processes. It was due to the fear that, if his words were taken as gospel by medical practitioners around the world, then the medical community might approach Ebola guinea with no mandate to truly comprehend this virus. Worse, they might perpetuate this misconception, causing others to trivialize the importance of understanding the potential functional significance of novel variants.

In fact, that was my precise experience: Others have gone further, to worsen the misinterpretation of the degree of genetic variation incorrectly. On the White House conference call, we were told, by a CDC scientist, that this strain was "well over 99.999% similar" to the strains from past *Zaire ebolavirus* disease outbreaks. I wrote to the scientist inquiring to see if they had been looking at different data. The *Zaire ebolavirus* isolate 1976 Yambuku-Mayinga (NC_002549.1) entry in National Center for Biotechnology

Information (NCBI) nucleotide database entry for has 18,959 base positions; the literature reports 396 differences; that's 97.9% similarity (not "well over 99.999%"). In evolutionary circles, this is called a "phenetic" difference; it measures the overall distance between strains, but does not inform at all on the biological, or evolutionary, significance of each individual difference. In Ebola circles, strains are recognized mostly by the degree of similarity to other strains. An unofficial cut-off of 10% seems generally accepted. However, this is a statistical, and not a biological, criterion for species demarcation. Given that the biology of *Ebolavirus* is so important to our survival, I recommend adopting a more holistic approach: We should consider clinical symptoms in light of the genetic distance, and not ignore potentially important clinical differences due to high genetic similarity.

At my niece's wedding in October, some of us were sitting around the table after the ceremony discussing current events. The discussion was centered on the politicization of the Ebola crisis, and I mentioned how politicians had asked the CDC director whether there were any mutations. One of my family members, Brian Murtagh, quipped:

> *It's funny how conservative politicians are, all of sudden, so concerned about evolution.*

The truth matters in all of science, always. With infectious disease, misrepresentation of the truth of evolution is dangerous. I am deeply concerned that, as result of assumption of the non-importance of the genetic variation, the necessary research to understand the potential significance of the mutations might be delayed, or worse, never take place. It is in evolutionary biology that we find the correct, albeit imperfect, set of lenses through which to view emerging infectious, and other, diseases. We have been dealt a hand of evolutionary heritage that provides us with a starting place from which to play this, and all future rounds. Technology may lift us beyond the innate capabilities that exist as part of that heritage, but our intelligence and abilities to create technology are also part of our evolutionary heritage. Perhaps ironically, evolutionary thinking drives our technology; many have used genetic algorithms to evolve solutions to complex problems, from algorithms for biomarker discovery to our current efforts at evolving antibody-like binding molecules and amplifiers that would allow the earliest possible detection of *Ebolavirus* in body fluids.

When I was an undergraduate student, my interest in research came to life when I attended, in the same semester, a course in genetics and a course in human evolution. At the time, the question of the fate of the Neanderthals was still very much a matter of speculation: Did we kill them, breed with them, or even eat them? The genetic data now tells us that not only did *Homo sapiens* breed with our human cousin *Homo neanderthalis*, we also incorporated genetic diversity from our other cousins, the Denisovans. We also know that it is very likely that the rich genetic diversity in our HLA genes is due, in part, to our absorption of the Neanderthal and other human genomes into the lineage that represents the cosmopolitan "us" today. HLA genes encode cell-surface antigen-presenting proteins, and the increased diversity affords us the ability to response to an amazing diversity of pathogens. While any speculation on what this might say about our character as a species is risky, I like to think that it points to the best characteristics of complex psychological make-up, innate capabilities, and tendencies. Genetically speaking, at least, we didn't leave them behind.

Also during my undergraduate years, DNA–DNA hybridization techniques were coming into vogue for use in studying evolutionary relationships among birds. In DNA–DNA hybridization, DNA from two species are isolated, and combined. In those studies, pioneered by Charles Sibley and Jon Edward Ahlquist, the DNAs from the two species were combined, and "melted," causing the hydrogen bonds to break in the native DNAs. The combined samples were then fused, or "annealed," at a lower temperature, and then re-melted. Some of the annealing occurred between the two species' DNAs, and the temperature at which the second melting took place was a key indicator of the overall genetic similarity between the two species. I had realized that the model for

calculating the distance made the assumption that the base com-
positions were the same for any pair of species. In reality, if they
were AT-rich, the melting temperature would be lower, and they
would appear to be less closely related. If they were GC-rich,
they would appear to more similar, and thus closely related.
Essentially, the unspecified model assumed that the cost of each
uncoupled nucleotide was equal, which, obviously, is not the case.
This idea was validated during a phone call to Vince Sarich, who
was at UC Berkeley at the time, to discuss the mathematical
assumptions   behind   the   DNA–DNA   hybridization-based
evolutionary distances. Vince was a gentlemanly scholar, took the
news well, congratulated me on my finding, and encouraged me to
pursue graduate studies. I am forever grateful for his objectivity.

A very positive possible outcome of this Ebola crisis would be if
more people came to appreciate the truly fundamental role that
evolution plays in determining our genetic ability to maintain our
well-being. While it has provided the basic building blocks we have
to work with, it has not constrained the solutions we can develop.
The restrictions that we place on ourselves, on the other hand, via
politics, dogma and doctrine could very well place restrictions on
our society's ability to cope with challenges posed to us by our
environment. We have both positive, and negative tendencies, but
they make us who we are. We have many "hang-overs" from our
Pleistocene ancestors, such as tribalism (which can be hijacked as
nationalism, or political "discourse"), sometimes with tragic consequences, such as war. We have a tendency to be concerned only
about events that directly affect us, and those we know or love, and
a tendency to hold onto to that which we know in favor of new
knowledge. These tendencies also cause us to lovingly care for our
family members, take pride in being part of community, and make
sacrifices for the greater good.

Contrary to most writings, evolution by natural selection is not
a "process"; rather, it is an outcome from a set of sufficient and
necessary circumstances: The existence of genetic variation tied to
differences in the ability of individuals to survive and reproduce.
This distinction between outcome and process is an important one

that goes well beyond semantics: If evolution is an outcome, then it, as an entity, cannot be juxtaposed against intelligent design. Evolution does not create in the directed sense that a Creator would create via his or her will; rather, evolution occurs.

Contrary to most representations, there also is no such force as "selective pressure"; evolution either occurs with, or without significance to the fitness of the individual. If gene frequencies change in a manner that is causally linked to the organisms' ability to survive, or reproduce, we call this "selection" (Darwin, 1859). In Charles Darwin's time, the molecular processes that determine an organism's many characteristics were unknown. Darwin used the term "natural selection" because he was attributing changes to organisms to the same general procedure that farmers were using at the time to change the characteristics of their crops and livestock. In the case of artificial selection, the farmer's choice to favor one phenotype over another is the factor that determines the direction of change; however, it is never thought of as a "force." The analogy of the environment "selecting" does not invoke intelligence, but, rather, provides the link between biological characteristics and their contribution to the survival and the relative reproduction of the individual expressing them.

Under Motoo Kimura's neutral theory of molecular evolution (Kimura, 1983), most (that is, mathematically most) changes in allele frequencies that occur do so by chance because the mutations have no particular significance to the survival or reproduction of individuals. This is, in large part, due to the nature of the genetic code: Nearly all third positions in a codon are "degenerate," or only lead to synonymous substitutions, which do not change the amino acid; many first position changes are also synonymous. However, most second positions do lead to amino acid changes that can alter the encoded protein's function. I do not see neutral theory as a criticism of natural selection: I find them to be complementary.

Criticism in science is valuable, because, like natural selection, it leads to improvements. The culture of science today, however, is, in places, corrupted by the view that criticism is "controversy." Authority seems to rule over data, not the other way around.

Vibrant, energetic discussions are healthy. They are necessary to produce understanding. Honest and frank sharing of competing views should set the tone for interactions among scientists, and with the public. Even as competitive as science has become, we must retain the ability to learn with, and from each other. The flaws in our thinking, and the flaws in our scientific processes, must be brought forward and dealt with frankly and honestly if we are to achieve the maximum benefit from society's investment in scientific infrastructure. Cherished notions and old habits that render misleading results must be subject to scrutiny. I have struggled with the field of gene expression's inability and unwillingness to grapple with the existence of a mathematical bias inherent to fold-change as a measure for differential expression in high-dimensional genomic and proteomic studies. In microarray studies, or whole transcriptome studies (i.e., RNA-seq), the expression of tens of thousands of genes is studied at the same time, and differences between clinical groups (e.g., tumor vs. normal) have, historically, been expressed as ratios. We have known for years that this approach is biased, and leaves out many genes from the analysis. Difference measures (e.g., tumor-normal) are more robust. The error in the common use of fold-change practice is unseen to most, and has, in my view, done more to hamper translational progress in biomedical research than any of the budget cuts to the NIH budget. After millions of dollars are spent on building research buildings, millions more on purchasing the latest technologies in genomics and proteomics, millions more spent on running studies to generate precious data on all types of disease, the use of fold-change to measure differential expression effectively results in throwing away large portions of the measurements. These observations are not a matter of personal preference; the method has dire consequences on the results. It's like a broken prism in a space telescope: We must deal with the truth to use our research tools effectively, even if it impeaches our past efforts, findings, preferences, and policy. Otherwise, we do harm to translational research and waste research resources, time, and lives.

We must not lose the benefits of the process of the generation of new ideas and new data, and the free and open discussion of their merits and weaknesses, and the impact they can have on our understanding of the universe, including ourselves. We see these flaws clearly through the lenses that Ebola has given us. It has provided us with lessons that apply to all areas of biomedical research.

If we are to reap the benefits of basic, clinical, and translational research, we need an era of progressive biomedical science in which assumptions are questioned, new questions are asked, and new answers are whole heartedly welcomed, and eyes don't roll when one proposes to make a difference in the clinic.

References

Darwin C. (1859) *On the Origin of Species by Means of Natural Selection, or the Preservation of Favoured Races in the Struggle for Life.* London, J. Murray.

Kimura M. (1983) *The Neutral Theory of Molecular Evolution.* Cambridge University Press, Cambridge.

9

Promising Treatments

"Treatment" of disease outbreaks involves operations at three levels: The individual and hospital level, the transmission chain, and the region. Each of these levels has its individual set of priorities and needs. As Dr. Michael Osterholm describes efforts as Plans A, B and C, the goal of Plan A is to respond quickly to the isolation and treatment of individuals. This is evidently ineffective for this strain. As Dr. Osterholm pointed out in October 2014: *"There is no Plan B. Plan C (meaning a vaccine) is many months away."*

Many have observed that people treated for EVD in the US have a much better outcome. There have been too few cases in the US for a significant result in any formal outcomes analysis; however, if this difference is real, it can perhaps be attributed in part to an overall healthier population, better nutrition, and better standards of treatment. Also, younger patients appear to do much better than older patients, for unknown reasons. Ebola survivor Dr. Kent Brantly of Samaritan's Purse knew this, which is why he suggested that his colleague receive the first of two available doses of Zmapp™.

Still, there are few direct treatments for EVD.

One of the most critical steps is to hydrate the patient. Health care workers in Africa use whatever means necessary. According to Dr. Gavin MacGregor-Skinner, Gatorade, even Coca-Cola have been used. He wondered, with a laugh, if these companies might provide more financial aid if they knew that their products were so critical in the fight at the frontlines.

The massive amounts of liquid waste, and the associated solid waste from each patient, made me wonder if doctors routinely treated patients for diarrhea, or if they saw that as part of the natural course of the disease. Treatments such as Imodium are not used, but the doctors have been successful in bringing down the fever with Tylenol. Proper hydration is thought to be key, although there is not yet consensus on the use of IVs in rural areas in Africa, and outcomes are better in the US, where dialysis and ventilators are available at the point of care.

Survivors of EVD have donated plasma in the hope that their antibodies will kick-start the immune response of new cases. To produce both humoral and cellular immune responses, serum and plasma from convalescent patients is sometimes used. During an outbreak of EVD in Kikwit, Democratic Republic of the Congo, transfusions from five convalescent patients to eight critically ill patients exhibiting symptoms reversed the course of the disease in all but one patient. Some of the patients were at the hemorrhagic stage, and two were comatose.

Vaccine Development

Immediate isolation of the sick, safe burial of the dead, and vaccination are seen as the highest public health priorities. There are some complexities to treatments such as the use of vaccines to boost an immune response. Under the Public Readiness and Emergency Preparedness (PREP) Act of 2005, The US Federal Government has provided immunity from prosecution for at least three promising vaccines (McCarthy, 2014).

The Center for Infectious Disease Research and Policy at the University of Minnesota has created, with the Wellcome Trust, a "Team B" consortium of experts who, in mid-January 2015, published a "Team B" document (Team B, 2015). This document, which will be revised over time, outlines the team's views on an awareness of changes in the epidemiology and ecology of the disease and the virus, calls for sustained funding for *Ebolavirus* research and for community engagement in the fight against EVD. They also call for close ethics and regulatory oversight of vaccine trials, studies designed to identify potential markers of successful protection (serologic correlates of protection). They provide a list of desiderata for vaccines for use in epidemics, including an extensive "Optimal and Minimal Criteria for Ebola Vaccines." Their treatment touches on many dimensions of practical concerns: What are we to do if success with one vaccine has the unfortunate effect of reducing enthusiasm for bringing forward other candidates? How do we know when protection has been achieved? They propose using unapproved vaccines in the clinical setting for the sake of helping to bend the curve, erstwhile conducting numerous trials of various sizes and forms, determined by practical local conditions.

Recall the sGP protein, one of the proteins encoded by the glycoprotein gene GP. While GP forms a three-part protein (trimer) with two differ forms of protein (Gp1 and Gp2) that together mediate cell entry, sGP plays an integral part of the *Ebolavirus'* attempts to thwart the immune system. sGP seems to inactivate neutrophils (Sullivan *et al.*, 2003), which are a small, highly mobile type of white blood cell in the immune system. They act as first-responders at the first sign of infection.

A study in the mouse revealed that an immune response to *Ebolavirus* was absent in mice that did not receive a sGP primer, which seemed to activate the overall immune response to *Ebolavirus*. Thus, it might be safer, and more informative, to conduct a study of vaccine with sGP, GP1GP2, alone compared to vaccine with sGP followed with a GP1GP2 vaccine, rather than vaccine vs. placebo. A Phase 1 clinical vaccine trial of 20 healthy volunteers showed that a chimpanzee adenovirus vector looks promising; positive reactions in volunteers show the production of neutralizing antibodies with minor side effects (Ledgerwood *et al.*, 2014).

In addition to prophylactic use, vaccines can be used as therapy to treat EVD. Johnson & Johnson has entered Phase I clinical trials of a vaccine called AdVac/MVA-BN Filo. This two-injection procedure uses a booster shot from the Danish company Bavarian Nordic to prime the immune system. This technique uses one form of the GP protein in the booster, and a second cocktail of

GP peptides representative of various strains of *Ebolavirus* in the second shot. Given positive results from an initial 20 human volunteers, and the durability of the protection provided by the two-shot approach found in the chimpanzee trial (Legderwood *et al.*, 2014), it is hoped that this technique will lead to hundreds of thousands of doses in early 2015 and millions of doses in late 2015.

Studies of a cocktail of antigens called ZMAb were found to cure infected monkeys of EVD, and to provide sustained protection against re-infection (Qui *et al.*, 2013). A third monoclonal antibody was added to ZMAb to create ZMapp™, a polyclonal antibody. This was the "secret serum" that was used by Dr. Brantly, and is very much in high demand. Not only can the vaccine be an effective prophylactic; there is every reason to expect that, if administered early enough, it can provide a curative treatment for EVD. Large-scale production of ZMapp™ is expected in 2015.

Another polyclonal antibody, developed from horse antibodies, is being developed in Japan by Vical Incorporated and AnGes MG. This equine polyclonal antibody therapy uses a DNA vaccine encoding an Ebola virus glycoprotein. In an early-stage clinical trial in 2014 of an experimental Ebola vaccine made by GlaxoSmithKline and the US NIAID, an immune response was found in all 20 healthy volunteers with no serious side effects. The study had two arms: A low dose one and a high dose one. This vaccine has components designed to protect against both *Sudan* and *Zaire ebolavirus*. The volunteers in the high dose arm showed a stronger immune response. Two types of T-cells were found to be elicited by the vaccine. In January 2015, this vaccine was found to have an "acceptable safety profile" by the WHO in Phase I trials.

A similar approach has been attempted by the US Army Medical Research Institute of Infectious Diseases (USAMRIID); they used VLPs (virus-like particles) made to express a combination of protein representing a wider range of Filoviruses, including *Ebolavirus*, Sudan virus, and Marburg virus. Their approach was to construct VLPs that express the sequence of Marburg GP2 in combination with a hybrid GP1 representative of *Ebolavirus* and *Sudan virus* GP sequences. Animal tests with guinea pigs resulted in strong cross-virus antibody production (Martins, 2015). In particular, they found that both GP2 and the C terminal region of GP1 are highly immunogenic.

A study of recombinant vesicular stomatitis virus (VSV) in 2008 (Geisbert *et al.*, 2008) showed that a modified VSV made to express *Zaire ebolavirus* glycoprotein Gp1 conferred complete immunity to *Ebolavirus* delivered to primates in a droplet chamber. The monkeys' heads were enclosed in a glass box, and they were exposed to mists of water containing *Zaire ebolavirus*. The result was that the exposure had been shown to cause no infections in 12 cynomolgus macaques (*Macaca fascicularis*) who had been vaccinated with the modified VSV. Control animals who were not vaccinated died from EVD.

Trials of the vaccine rVSV-ZEBOV (Merck and New Link Genetics) were halted temporarily due to joint pain side effects in some of the participants. rVSV-ZEBOV, which carries the strain's glycoprotein coding sequence in the genome of a vesicular stomatitis virus, has been proven effective against the Zaire strain in the crab-eating macaque (Geisbert *et al.*, 2008). Those trials resumed in January 2015, and rVSV-ZEBOV was also given the green-light on WHO safety in January 2015.

Pharmaceutical Hopefuls

Zmapp™, manufactured by Mapp Biopharmaceutical, is an experimental drug that includes mouse antibodies to three Ebola proteins. In such medicines, antibodies are harvested from mice who had not been exposed to the virus itself, but rather to fragments of Ebola proteins (peptides). In the case of Zmapp™, the protein sequence was determined from the mouse experiments, and then the peptides are grown in plants.

The drug, which had shown promise to reverse the disease in non-human primate trials (Qiu *et al.*, 2014), was first used on humans under a compassionate use protocols. The two patients it was used on were US citizens, Dr. Kent Brantly and Nancy Writebol. Dr. Brantly and Writebol were in Liberia on a mission of mercy with the organization Samaritan's Purse. They fell ill with Ebola; on the ninth day of symptoms, two doses of Zmapp™ arrived from San Diego, CA; Dr. Brantly requested that his colleague be given the first dose. However, as his condition suddenly worsened, and Dr. Brantly felt as if he were dying, he requested the first dose. While the FDA has reservations over the attribution of Dr. Brantly's survival to Zmapp™, those present at the time describe it as a complete reversal: The drug appeared to reverse final stage EVD in Dr. Brantly. His transformation was remarkable; within hours of receiving his single dose, his rash subsided, his temperature reduced, and he was ambulatory upon reaching the US days later. Writebol was given the second dose, and she also recovered.

According to the strictures of science, the level of evidence required to actually attribute their survival to Zmapp™ is a properly controlled clinical study. Dr. Brantly may have been given a better standard of care than most others in Africa, and he had been given plasma from a teenage male patient he had previously treated. He only showed reversal after Zmapp™ was administered, so his reversal arguably should be attributed to Zmapp™, not to the standard of care. However, larger studies are the classically accepted type of data. We technically cannot ascribe his survival to Zmapp™, but descriptions of the reversal of his symptoms are compelling.

Research on live *Ebolavirus* requires a BSL4 laboratory. A major potential step forward was made by researchers. Dr. John McKew and Dr. Wei Zheng, working at the National Center for Advancing Translational Sciences, an arm of the National Institutes of Health, called Dr. Adolfo Garcia-Sastre with an idea. They had seen his team's work from a few years ago where he and colleagues had design a surrogate "mimic" assay that could be used outside of biocontainment to test for vaccines and drugs. They had developed a virus-like particle (VLP) that had some of the capability of two highly pathogenic viruses: Ebola and a high pathogenic influenza strain. Adolfo's *Ebolavirus* mimic is a virus core that has the Gp1Gp2-mediated host cell entry mechanism only; it does not contain any of the other genes, so the VLP is harmless and can be used in any lab.

During their phone call, the NIH compound group lead scientists informed Adolfo that they had libraries of compounds of FDA-approved drugs, some of which might be shown to inhibit the mimic's ability to enter human tissues.

Together, Adolfo's team tried over 2,800 compounds in one screen. They found 53 that had significant ability to inhibit the VLP's entry into human cells in culture (Kouznetsova *et al.*, 2014). I spoke with Adolfo in late December. Many compounds showed high cytotoxicity and selectivity, and many were anticancer drugs. He said it was remarkable the short amount of time to set up the assay to the optimization of the screen.

> *From the time they called me until the screening was finished was only a few months. The fit between their compound resource and our move into high-throughput screening was perfect. It was a great fit, and I'm very happy with the outcome.*

I asked Adolfo if the screens had been done with the Gp1Gp2 protein sequences from Ebola guinea. He told me that the screen was done with *Zaire ebolavirus*, not the actual outbreak strain, but that would be important only if the virus were to change the fundamental function of entry, such as change of a target receptor. Under those conditions, some modes of entry may be missed, but Adolfo thinks that it is very unlikely to have occurred in Ebola guinea. None of the areas of the GP gene found to be important for the Zmapp™ activity harbor amino acid altering substitutions (Dr. Erica Ollman, *pers. comm.*). I asked Aldofo what the focus of the future of his research was; he said they are hard at work screening additional compounds, in search of one initially that will shut down Ebola guinea. In the long run, he said ideally they would like to discovery compounds that can inhibit most, if not all, *Ebolavirus* strains.

Although all of the compounds tested have been FDA-approved, Adolfo expects that, unfortunately, it will take longer to get FDA approval; he expects the next steps will involve live virus testing and then animal model, prior to human studies. The human studies may also have to determine optimal doses.

For example, while some compounds have been approved for cancer, the toxicity may be too much in the context of EVD.

Adolfo's VLP mimic only uses Gp1Gp2. I was curious about the other genes, and whether his team was planning studies of mimics of other functions. He said:

> *In addition to host cell entry, replication is important, so RNA polymerase activity could be mimicked, as well as the function of genes that inhibit innate immune response, such as interferon inhibitors. Other groups are using this; RNA mimic that encodes a reporter gene with EBV RNA polymerase promoters but instead of the viral genes, it has reporters.*

I wondered out loud if antisense RNAs could be incorporated into the RNA mimic, a sort of gene therapy. Antisense RNA is the reverse complement of the RNA that encodes a protein; it is used to silence the expression of genes, usually in cell lines, to determine the functional or effects of the loss of gene. Adolfo liked the idea, and said:

> *Gene therapy is another perfectly reasonable option, however, in EVD, the challenge would be to be able to introduce it into enough cells to be effective. Small drugs, by comparison, are easy to penetrate.*

This is a very promising development, as some of these drugs are no doubt readily available and could be used in rapid trials. Our conversation continued on to some of the other pressing issues. Adolfo, like so many involved in research on *Ebolavirus*, is humane in his thinking about priorities:

> *You know, Jim, an outbreak like the one that happened has been predicted (sooner or later), and we are far worse off than we could have been because between outbreaks, there has been a great deal of complacency. It is critically important to realize a lesson to be learned about zoonotic viruses; they are constantly jumping to humans, and it was only a matter of time before one took off. We need to keep research on*

these pathogens going, and we should make studies of transmission modalities a priority.

The question of treatment/placebo clinical trials with a disease as deadly as EBV is a weighty one. For years, I admired the work of clinical researchers and others working in support of biomedical research who would opt to change the protocol for patients during the mid-course of a trial given early promising results. This is no small sacrifice for the validity of the science; in clinical studies, random allocation of patients to treatment groups is the gold standard by which the validity of the result of a study is measured. However, in the case of Ebola, individual responses to treatment such as Zmapp™ may be seen to reverse the course of the disease with visible results. Thus, some have called for initial trials to forego the placebo controls, allowing all patients the experimental treatment, and if a universal positive response is seen, then larger studies would follow to find the limits of the drug's efficacy, minimizing unnecessary human suffering. If such a study were to fail for a larger proportion of patients, the benefit could not be measured, and then a second, placebo-controlled study could be conducted in which patients were allocated to whichever therapy appeared most effective until the value of the treatment is clear (*New York Times*, Dec 1, 2014). Such adaptive designs are hard to interpret if there is a negative result because the power of the study is compromised and the analysis of the data becomes complicated. Nevertheless, a large number of small trials could be conducted: An initial foray.

Another option is treatment vs. treatment. Two or more experimental treatments may be used at random on patients in a trial, with the goal being to determine if there is a significant difference in their efficacy and long-term safety. For this kind of trial, existing baseline data from patients from the recent past who could not yet benefit from the novel treatments could be established. Confounding could be avoided using multivariate matching, a process in which baseline patients are chosen from a database of patients that match patients considering demographic and clinical variables (age, gender, parity, existing and past diagnosis, smoking history, etc.). In this manner, the studies could hopefully show that both experimental treatments were more effective than no treatment, and that both were safe and equally effective.

Favipiravir, designed for RNA influenza viruses, has been shown to be effective in an EVD mouse model (Oestereich *et al.*, 2014; Smither *et al.*, 2014). Various other compounds that have shown antiviral activities in early stage cell culture studies include a 1,7-bis(alkylamino)diazachrysene-based small molecule that had previously been shown to inhibit botulinum neurotoxin (Opsenica *et al.*, 2011). There may be hope for treatments.

Managing the Spread via "Ebola-Free Zones"

In late December 2014, WHO convened in Geneva for a discussion of the creation of "Ebola Resilience Capacity Zones" that, if successful, will be transformed into "Ebola Free Zones". This is an organizational principle that breaks the problem down into smaller, more manageable pieces. The idea of these zones is that it is simpler logistically to think of the overall problem in small, well-defined geographic areas than to try to do the impossible of managing all of the events that happen within a country or region. This strategy was used successfully in 2008 with the H1N5 influenza outbreaks in Egypt, Indonesia and Vietnam (MacGregor-Skinner, *pers. comm.*)

Treating the Reservoir Hosts

Convincing evidence is mounting that the reservoir includes various fruit-eating bat species. It is highly possible that bats attracted to palm tree plantations in Guinea brought the virus with them; if so, then the migratory patterns and dispersal patterns of these reservoir hosts should be thoroughly studied and considered. Seropositive bats have been found in the wild (Hayman *et al.*, 2012). *Ebolavirus* has been found to be shed in the feces of experimentally infected fruit bats for up to three weeks (Swanepoel *et al.*, 1996), and the closely related *Marburg virus* has been isolated in fruit bats (Towner *et al.*, 2009). Other evidence, specifically the distribution of antibodies in animals studied in the wild, suggests that the rain forest, from time to time, is teeming with animals with *Ebolavirus* (Gonzalez *et al.*, 2005). The virus also quite possibly could be a plant product that acts to fend off predation by animals, including bats: Ebola outbreaks also appear to occur following heavy rains after dry spells (Pinzon *et al.*, 2005; Tucker *et al.*, 2002).

One strategy that we might consider is to immunize fruit bats populations against *Ebolavirus* via sprayed fruits left high in trees, near their caves. Immunization of threatened and endangered wild animals to protect them from diseases has been successful in the past (Haydon *et al.*, 2006), and vaccination of wildlife against rabies is commonplace, but this is not without challenges, which could be learned from (Williams *et al.*, 2006; Rupprecht *et al.*, 2004). Although a study on intrathoracic inoculation of *Reston ebolavirus* failed to produce any evidence of viral replication in three mosquito species (Turell *et al.*, 1996), and a survey of the fauna in 1999 after the DRC outbreak (Reiter *et al.*, 1999) did not reveal a single *Ebolavirus* isolate from arthropods, possible vectors such as ticks and fleas should be tested for *ebolavirus*. The life cycle and zoonotic transmissions of Ebola are not completely known.

Hemopurification (Dialysis)

Deaths from EVD stem from the destruction of critical blood vessels and organs as the coagulopathy effects of the cytokine storm turn the body against itself. To reduce the cytokine storm, Aethlon Medical, Inc. created the Hemopurifier, which removes viruses, and sheds glycoproteins (the "flak" of Ebola's battle plan) and toxins from the blood of patients. The device apparently reversed the course of the disease in a Ugandan doctor EVD patient in Germany, who had progressed to the point of multiple organ failure, and it has been used successfully on nearly 100 HIV and Hepatitis C patients. The device is designed for use in standard Continuous Renal Replacement Therapy (CRRT) machines (dialysis). In early January 2015, the Aethlon Hemopurifier was approved by the FDA for testing on 20 EVD patients in the US. An in-depth description of the application of RRT on an EVD patient at Emory University is described by Connor *et al.*, (2015). It also includes detailed descriptions of safety protocols resulting in "no detectable *Ebolavirus* genetic material in the spent RRT effluent waste."

There are many good reasons for hope for effective treatments.

References

Connor MJ Jr, Kraft C, Mehta AK, *et al.* (2015) Successful delivery of RRT in Ebola virus disease. *J Am Soc Nephrol* **26(1):** 31–7. doi: 10.1681/ASN.2014111057. Epub Nov 14, 2014.

Geisbert TW, Daddario-Dicaprio KM, Geisbert JB, *et al.* (2008) Vesicular stomatitis virus-based vaccines protect nonhuman primates against aerosol challenge with Ebola and Marburg viruses. *Vaccine* **26(52):** 6894–900. doi: 10.1016/j.vaccine.2008.09.082.

Gonzalez JP, Herbreteau V, Morvan J, Leroy EM. (2005) Ebola virus circulation in Africa: a balance between clinical expression and epidemiological silence. *Bull Soc Pathol Exot* **98(3):** 210–7.

Haydon DT, Randall DA, Matthews L, *et al.* (2006) Low-coverage vaccination strategies for the conservation of endangered species. *Nature* **443(7112):** 692–5.

Hayman DTS, Yu M, Crameri G, *et al.* (2012) Ebola virus antibodies in fruit bats, Ghana, West Africa [letter]. *Emerg Infect Dis* [serial on the Internet]. [http://dx.doi.org/10.3201/eid1807.111654]

Kouznetsova J, *et al.* (2014) Identification of 53 compounds that block Ebola virus-like particle entry via a repurposing screen of approved drugs. *Emerg Microbes Infect* **3:** e84. doi:10.1038/emi.2014.88.

Ledgerwood JE, *et al.* (2014) Chimpanzee adenovirus vector Ebola vaccine — preliminary report. *N Engl J Med*, Nov 26, 2014. [http://www.nejm.org/doi/full/10.1056/NEJMoa1410863]

Martins K, Carra JH, Cooper CL, *et al.* (2014) Cross-protection conferred by filovirus virus-like particles containing trimeric hybrid glycoprotein. *Viral Immunol* **28(1):** 62–70. doi: 10.1089/vim.2014.0071.

McCarthy M. (2014) US provides immunity from legal claims related to three Ebola vaccines. *Br Med J* **349:** g7608. doi: 10.1136/bmj.g7608.

Oestereich L, Lüdtke, A, Wurr S, *et al.* (2014) Successful treatment of advanced Ebola virus infection with T-705 (favipiravir) in a small animal model. *Antiviral Res* **105:** 17–21. doi:10.1016/j.antiviral. 2014.02.014.

Opsenica I, Burnett JC, Gussio R, *et al.* (2011) A chemotype that inhibits three unrelated pathogenic targets: the botulinum neurotoxin serotype A light chain, P. falciparum malaria, and the Ebola filovirus. *J Med Chem* **54(5):** 1157–69. doi: 10.1021/jm100938u. Epub Jan 25, 2011.

Pinzon E, Wilson JM, Tucker CJ. (2005) Climate-based health monitoring systems for eco-climatic conditions associated with infectious diseases. *Bull Soc Pathol Exot* **98(3):** 239–43.

Qiu X, Audet J, Wong G, *et al.* (2013) Sustained protection against Ebola virus infection following treatment of infected nonhuman primates with ZMAb. *Sci Rep* **3:** 3365. doi: 10.1038/srep03365.

Qiu X, *et al.* (2014) Reversion of advanced Ebola virus disease in nonhuman primates with ZMapp. *Nature* **514(7520):** 47–53. doi: 10.1038/nature13777.

Reiter P, Turell M, Coleman R, *et al.* (1999) Field investigations of an outbreak of Ebola hemorrhagic fever, Kikwit, Democratic Republic of the Congo, 1995: arthropod studies. *J Infect Dis* **179(Suppl 1):** S148–54.

Rupprecht CE, Hanlon CA, Slate D. (2004) Oral vaccination of wildlife against rabies: opportunities and challenges in prevention and control. *Dev Biol (Basel)* **19:** 173–84.

Smither SJ, Eastaugh LS, Steward JA, *et al.* (2014) Post-exposure efficacy of oral T-705 (favipiravir) against inhalational Ebola virus infection in a mouse model. *Antiviral Res* **104:** 153–5. doi:10.1016/j.antiviral.2014.01.012

Sullivan N, Yang Z-Y, Naebl GJ. (2003) Ebola virus pathogenesis: implications for vaccines and therapies. *J Virol* **77:** 9733–37.

Swanepoel R, Leman PA, Burt FJ, *et al.* (1996) Experimental inoculation of plants and animals with Ebola virus. *Emerg Infect Dis* **2:** 321–325.

Team B. (2015) Fast-track development of ebola vaccines: principles and target product criteria. Jan 12, 2015. [http://www.cidrap.umn.edu/

sites/default/files/public/downloads/wellcome_trust-cidrap_ebola_ vaccine_team_b_interim_report-final.pdf]

Towner JS, Amman BR, Sealy TK, *et al.* (2009) Isolation of genetically diverse Marburg viruses from Egyptian fruit bats. *PLOS Pathog* **5(7):** e1000536. doi: 10.1371/journal.ppat.1000536.

Tucker CJ, Wilson JM, Mahoney R, *et al.* (2002) Climatic and ecological context of the 1994–1996 ebola outbreaks. *Photogram Eng Remote Sens* **68(2):** 144–52.

Turell MJ, Bressler DS, Rossi CA. (1996) Short report: lack of virus replication in arthropods after intrathoracic inoculation of Ebola Reston virus. *Am J Trop Med Hyg* **55(1):** 89–90.

Williams SD, Pollinger JP, Cleaveland S, *et al.* (2006) Low-coverage vaccination strategies for the conservation of endangered species. *Nature* **443(7112):** 692–5.

10

Policy Analysis

The US population is faced with apparently conflicting signals from government officials on the degree to which they should be concerned over the risks that the West African outbreak of Ebola Virus Disease (EVD) poses to the American public. The CDC's position on Ebola was that they were ready to deal with Ebola making it to the US; that mandatory quarantine is not necessary; that the risk of an outbreak here in the US is very low. They appeared confident that an outbreak will not occur in the US, and that we should not be overly concerned about the few cases that have made it to the US, nor of the few cases due to transmission to health care workers, and potential instances of transmission to loved one. These statements were at odds with the data coming out of Africa, and the information provided by the media. I am scientist; the logical basis of inferences is important to me. Dr. Anthony Fauci, director of the NIAID, and others, have been quoted as saying that we should base policy on science, not on fear. Some of the media and state government's reaction has been dismissed as "hysteria." However, fear may also exist within our species' genetically encoded hardware upon which the environment, including our parents, writes psychological software. The detect-and-fear repertoire capacity exists for a reason: It has contributed to our survival.

Young goslings are known to have innate fear of (well, aversion to, at least) silhouettes of larger birds of prey relative to non-prey bird forms: They crouch, or run in response to large, moving hawk shapes but have no such response when a goose form is flown

159

overhead (e.g., Canty and Gould, 1995). Our ancestors in our hominid lineage who did not fear predators and venomous animals may have been subject to increased mortality rates due to venom, parasites, and viral diseases such as rabies, and perhaps even viruses like Ebola.

Our instinctual reactions to certain objects in our environment has been documented; for example, infants as well as adults are able to detect figures of snakes better than other, more benign objects (LoBue and DeLoache, 2008). Dr. David Rakison is the director of the Infant Cognition Laboratory at Carnegie Mellon University. He uses gaze persistence in naive infants to test for evidence that we are hard-wired to be biased to study objects in our environment that might be dangerous to us. His studies have indicated that five-month old human infants may be pre-programmed to preferentially detect spiders in their environment compared to relatively benign objects (e.g., flowers and mushrooms; Rakison and Derringer, 2008). While we are not born "afraid" of spiders, we seem to have inherited a "perceptual template" for increased interest in the spider pattern. His results have been replicated using snake patterns. Our bias toward fear of spiders appears to be validated by a 2005 Gallup poll on fear, which reported spiders as the number two thing Americans fear.

While there is no reason why hominids, or mammals in general, could not have also evolved the ability to detect certain patterns in animal forms as an adaptation to living in a dangerous world, the question of nature vs. nurture arises. Don't we learn what to fear from our families, and our elders? I spoke with David about his studies and found out that there is more evidence in support of the existence of perceptual templates, and how we appear to use them. Further study showed that fear-learning, the ability to rapidly associate negative emotions to objects like spiders and snakes, based on visual facial cues in human faces, occurs. His studies showed, however, that no such response occurs with benign objects like flowers. He also found that the reaction that reflects fear-learning was found to occur in female, but not male, 11-month old infants (Rakison, 2009).

It may be no surprise to find that fear is learned, and males at a very young age may be less prone to associating with others' expression of fears to objects in the environment for which we have evolved perceptual templates. But these studies have implications for our understanding of social dynamics related to fear in response to the possibility of infectious outbreaks in America. First, the majority of Americans are utterly dependent on government officials for information about risks associated with contagious diseases as complex as EVD.

Second, given the large amount of mortality associated with contagious diseases, we almost certainly have something of a perception template for things that might harm us that we do not quite fully understand. The human mind seeks tirelessly to understand its environment, and, in the absence of facts, we either rely on our leaders for information, or we create stories as to the origins, and mechanisms, of the risk. So when the CDC came out with uncertainty, and, worse, with information that could not withstand even a modest amount of scrutiny, the public trust was partly lost.

It would be interesting to see if infants react similarly to images of organisms that are associated with increased risk of infectious diseases, and if variation exists across cultures in response to local venomous animals.

On top of this potential genetic background for detection of potential dangers, it is well known in behavioral psychology circles that genetic variation exists within genes associated with risk-taking and novelty-seeking, such as the dopamine D4 receptor (Ebstein *et al.*, 1996; Benjamin *et al.*, 1996).

Fear provides a healthy balance for those who otherwise might take unnecessary and unwise risks. Fear alone can do no harm; it's just an emotion. What we do with our fear is of the utmost importance. If we act rashly, we may harm ourselves or others. If we act responsibly, then we can remain rational about our fears. If we respect ourselves and accept that we humans are products of our rich evolutionary heritage, we can see that our fears can also be of immense value: They can mobilize hundreds, or thousands of people willing to make donations, make sacrifices, and donate time packaging supplies bound for Western Africa. Fear is a tool for use in a crisis. Bravery is defined as doing what needs to be done in the face of fear of acknowledged risk. Every time a health care worker dons their PPG in preparation for their treatment or tending of a patient with EVD, they may be afraid, but more importantly, they are being brave. Every time a bioinformatician shares the unfortunate bad news of poor data quality, or a biostatistician shares news of a confounding variable in a study design with their peers, they are being brave. Truth in science matters, and even if it is an unfortunate or uncomfortable truth, it must be told. There can be consequences that result from bearing bad news to people who might wish otherwise, who might wish to "spin" their results as favorably as possible.

(In science and technology), reality must take precedence over public relations, for nature cannot be fooled.

— Richard Feynman, 1986.

Science provides a respite from the spin; it is meant to provide a truly objective viewpoint. To attempt to modulate how we feel about a scientific topic should not be any government official's aim. Good science requires that we divorce our subjective feelings from the logic of the interpretation of the data. This is not always easy to do, but it is necessary. Government officials are entrusted with the public health; their job, however, is not to tell us how to feel about something that might affect our lives, but rather, to provide us with the facts and to tell us what we need to know so that we can decide how to act responsibly. It does not engender public trust when a dire situation is sugar-coated, and when the best-case scenario does not manifest, mistrust and suspicion results. Speaking with both professionals and lay persons in my life, i.e., those not involved in scientific research or biomedical practice, I've learned that the attempts by the CDC to assuage the fears of American public about the Ebola crisis were seen broadly as just not believable, especially during the House Oversight hearings just prior to the mid-term elections. In conversations with waitresses, a plumber, and a truck driver, shortly after the testimony, I learned that their shared impression was that the CDC was obviously hiding something; that "they" (i.e., the CDC) did not want the American public to know "how bad it was." Why would the general public get that impression? Some people toyed with radical, non-sensical conspiracy theories ("Ebola is population control," somehow related to the so-called "Georgia Guidestones"), but some did wonder if I thought the government wanted a massive die-off. One person I spoke with cited what she saw as blatant racism. "It's okay if blacks in Africa die by the thousands," she said. "But get one white doctor sick, and the entire media lights up — they pull out all the stops, use the experimental medicines. These people should be investigated," she quipped.

Perhaps a dose of fear is, from an evolutionary viewpoint at least, rational. Most would call this type of rational fear "respect." Professor Peter Piot, who is best known as part of the team who discovered the Ebola virus, was quoted as having said:

In 1976, I discovered Ebola — now I fear an unimaginable tragedy. Around June it became clear to me there was something different about this outbreak. I began to get really worried.

— *The Guardian, 6, Oct 2014*

Bravery is not the absence of fear. It is the ability to do the right thing, the hard thing, in spite of being afraid in the face of possible negative consequences. Adrenaline increase caused by fear can increase our focus; it enhances our ability to sequester new information into long-term memory. Being afraid of Ebola is not automatically the same thing as being irresponsible. If the government's goal was to modulate the public's perception so they are less reactionary, well, that would be irresponsible. If, or when, the truth comes out, or if things just happen to get worse, then the officials would have lost legitimacy with the public, and the public would start to wonder what else they were being lied to about that might also be a threat to them. We should not ignore our evolutionary heritage, especially in circumstances where the fate of millions of lives is potentially at stake. Even if we all agreed on the interpretation of the evidence, our individual subjective risk preferences would still cause disagreements on the degree of importance to assign each factor. The oft-stated mantra that public health policy should only ever be founded on science, and not on fear, should not preclude a thorough, passionate concern for the well-being of the population, weighing the risks to the few against the benefits to the many. At times the call to not be motivated by fear seems to be missing an altogether human component. This is one of those times.

It will be perhaps useful, therefore, to examine the rational basis (or lack thereof) of the many statements produced in support of one or another message during this time. Some are, in fact, logically supported, while some include a smattering of subjective, non-science-based policy due to omissions, selective use of scientific data, or even misrepresentation of the published data. As the goal is to increase understanding, and not point to fingers or place blame, these positions are perhaps best considered "unresolved," as opposed to "wrong."

The types of statements that appear to have the effect of increasing, however incrementally, the risk of transmission are especially concerning; for the most part, they appear as universal statements encompassing all conditions, without exception. It was, I think, these types of unqualified statements that did not mesh with expectations. Certain logic flaws may also currently place the US population at unnecessary risk to infection via spread of the *Ebolavirus*, and if the same logic flaws are in play in the EVD health care policies in Africa, one wonders if they may be helping to unwittingly drive the epidemic in West Africa.

Probabilities and Modes of Transmission

The most pressing original question on the *Ebolavirus* outbreak to people in the US was: "What is possibility of someone in the US acquiring EVD?" That possibility is known and, expressed as a probability, is 100%. We know that the virus is highly virulent, and at late stages, highly infectious. So the probability seems high independent of any data. We have some observational data, however — the type that the FDA does not want to be used in clinical trials for drugs: The two nurses who became infected represent the first human–human transmission of *Ebolavirus* in the US. Thus, their cases are data that inform us about the possibility of transmission overall: The probability is 1.0.

A natural secondary question is: "What is the probability that an individual in the US will become infected with *Ebolavirus*?"

This answer to this question is also knowable, and the answer is a function of the number of cases that currently exist in the US and the rate and possible modes of transmission of *Ebolavirus.*

The possible modes of transmission are universally represented as:

Person-to-person transmission is possible due to contact with body fluids from an Ebola-infected person showing symptoms of EBV.

As Dr. Anthony Fauci stated on Sunday, Oct 19, 2014:

I can just tell you that what we want to do is to make sure first, protect the American public, but do so based on scientific data, where we keep repeating over and over again, the scientific data tells us that people who are without symptoms, with whom you don't come into contact with body fluids, are not a threat, they will not get infected.

Note the dual conditions here in this statement. It means, more concisely:

If you do not come into contact with body fluids from people who have symptoms, you will not get infected.

This statement does not address whether this mode of transmission is the exclusive mode of transmission; to be fair, one has to take the statements in the full context of all of the other statements available. But we'll get to indirect transmission in a moment.

Dr. Fauci also stated, more assertively:

As we have said many times, people without symptoms do not transmit Ebola. We know that. So, guidelines regarding how you handle people from coming back should always be based on the science. And science tells us that people who are asymptomatic do not transmit.

Basically, the official medical position is that transmission can only occur from infected people who are sick (symptomatic).

These statements, unfortunately, are not based on scientific data from human subjects. All of the data cited by the CDC's position (CDC, 2014) are clinical observational data, citing the absence of transmissions *that can be ascribed* to indirect transmission. The basis of this knowledge claim depends on the *absence of data;* specifically that none of the transmissions that have occurred with this new strain have been proven to involve pre-symptomatic transmission. Recall that drug companies cannot bring to market drugs whose safety and efficacy are based exclusively on animal studies. If we apply the same standard, the same level of evidence, to this aspect of policy as the FDA would require of all Ebola drug trials, we have to see that there have been no properly controlled studies that indicate that transmission between infected humans and non-infected humans is impossible. Naturally, such studies would be terribly unethical: *No one should ever be subjected unnecessarily to infection with Ebolavirus or to risk of death from EVD.* An important question is: Have there been any instances in which people come down with EBV without knowingly coming into contact with an EBV patient with symptoms?

In fact, transmission to health care workers from undiagnosed, infected people may very well be occurring in cryptic ways, especially, for example, if they are treating patients for non-Ebola conditions that involve intimate care (blood samples, for example). Take, for example, the case of Thomas Eric Duncan. He was misdiagnosed, and thus, officially, he was not diagnosed with EVD. The nurses and other hospital staff were fully exposed to him as a regular patient. Duncan exhibited symptoms, and stated he had traveled from West Africa (and that the attending physician missed this point). Fast forward to a point in the future (which we hope never occurs) in which there are hundreds or thousands of cases of Ebola in the US. People with the flu, with broken arms, etc., may present no symptoms of Ebola, and yet the probability of transmission exists due to viremia. Although transmission is most likely during the end stages of the disease, when patients have the highest viremia, it takes, in principle, just one copy of *Ebolavirus* (i.e., a single virion) to transmit the disease from one person to another. In spite of all of the observational data, no evidence from properly controlled clinical trials exist that would allow us to rule out that person-to-person transmission is possible due to contact with body fluids from a person infected with *Ebolavirus* without symptoms of EVD.

The following scenarios do not seem unlikely, and even if they are rare, they should be a concern if there is a large epidemic underway:

— An asymptomatic person infected with *Ebolavirus* is being treated for a non-EVD condition, causing health care workers (HCWs) to unknowingly come into contact with body fluids from an infected person
— An asymptomatic man infected with *Ebolavirus* has unprotected sex with another person
— An asymptomatic person infected with *Ebolavirus* donates blood, and it is not screened for *Ebolavirus*.

On day 1 (exposure), the probability of transmission must be near zero; at death, and afterwards, the person is extremely contagious, and the probability of transmission (if the body is touched) must be near certainty. What the curve of the probability of transmission actually looks like from infection, through incubation, to death must be estimated. Estimates of the infectious period range from 5–8 days, Most people become symptomatic between 8 and 10 days after infection, whereas most patients die between 6 and 15 days from the onset of symptoms, depending on the reference. Some cases, however, progress immediately, and some do not progress until late in the 21-day period. The likelihood of asymptomatic transmission may be very low, but logic dictates that it should be related to the concentration of viruses in the blood of patients (viremia); viral growth is logarithmic in asymptomatic people; thus the risk should increase the closer one comes to symptoms. The claim of zero probability of transmission before symptoms, if wrong, would be tragic. If people are contagious prior to symptoms, becoming increasingly contagious as viremia increases, it could help explain the high number of transmissions to, and perhaps among, health care workers.

The often-repeated, unqualified position that one can become infected only via direct contact with body fluids from an infected person implies that these other possibilities (and others) are not a source for concern. There are risks in these scenarios that cannot be anticipated and are ignored by the overarching statements that infection cannot occur from people without symptoms. The probability may be small, especially in the initial stages of an epidemic when the number of patients is small. That small probability exists in each infected patient for around 21 days. The probability of such transmissions, as a regular occurrence, approaches 1.0 at epidemic numbers, especially in dense populations, and thus should be allowed as possible future cause of grave concern. The lack of such qualifiers in the statements from the CDC and the NIH increases future risk, and their positions may update given new data. However small the probability, the probability that any given number of these kinds of events will occur in a given region increases as the number of cases increase.

The CDC website also includes the statement:

> *Ebola is spread through direct contact ... with objects (like needles and syringes) that have been contaminated with the virus.*

There are additional objects that seem important to consider. The question of whether one could become infected via objects such as via shared towels (as in methicillin-resistant *Staphylococcus aureus* (MRSA) transmission), or shared toothbrushes and dentist drills (as in in 1990s case of Florida HIV transmission) is not addressed. We are not transferring what we have learned from other diseases to Ebola. However, we know that the *Ebolavirus* is known to be in high concentrations in saliva at the earliest stages of the disease. And we know its concentration in saliva tracks viremia in the blood very closely.

The number of incidental MRSA infections that occur due to indirect infections in the US is estimated at over 79,000 patients per year. The durability of MRSA on fomites can be as high as eight weeks (Desai *et al.*, 2011). According to the Material Safety Data Sheet (MSDS) on Ebola, and the Canadian Pathogen Safety Data Sheet (see full quotes in Chapter 4), the durability is a number of days, or weeks, depending on conditions. If indirect MRSA transmission leads to over 70,000 cases per year, and can survive eight weeks on surfaces outside of the body, the number of indirect transmission cases expected per year for *Ebolavirus* is, for various estimates from the scientific literature:

Fomite	Time	Expected # of Cases/Yr
Surface	"days" (assume 3)	3,750
Blood	"weeks" (assume 2)	17,500
Dried on glass	50 days	62,500

It seems highly unlikely that the CDC and the NIH would ever find, at anytime, 3,750 to 17,500 Ebola indirect transmissions in the US per year to be an "acceptable risk." The question of whether MRSA transmission rates provide a good model for Ebola is an important one, but whatever the best model, the expected numbers are not zero. Their statements amount to: "Life can proceed as normal until someone has symptoms"; this ignores conditions under which people can be exposed to risk of infection in spite of the absence of symptoms. The risk may be perceived to be small; however, pre-symptomatic transmission is a logical route to a large outbreak, under the right conditions, and therefore the public should be highly concerned over persons exposed to Ebola-positive patients.

The large number of cases that report during interview no known exposure to symptomatic persons is also a potential indication of indirect transmission. Indirect transmission, or asymptomatic transmission, could explain the case of the patient who brought Ebola from Monrovia to Nigeria (he reported no contact with anyone with the illness; Shaib *et al.*, 2014). One incident of transmission via shared blanket has been reported (Francesconi *et al.*, 2003). Perhaps the safest assumption to make is that someone who has flu symptoms may infect loved ones and others with *Ebolavirus* via indirect transmission, and precautions should be taken.

The CDC website statement "You CAN'T get Ebola through FOOD grown or legally purchased in the U.S." appears to ignore the observation made in 2007 by the authors of a study published in the *Journal of Infectious Diseases* (Bausch *et al.*, 2007):

> *Of particular concern is the frequent presence of EBOV in saliva early during the course of disease, where it could be transmitted to others through intimate contact and from sharing food, especially given the custom, in many parts of Africa, of eating with the hands from a common plate.*

While the CDC's statement may be correct, we can conclude that Ebola can be transmitted by *sharing* food and plates. Bushmeat from Africa is sold illegally in some markets in the US.

The CDC information can be seen to be misleading because it seems to make a universal claim, without qualification, and it fails to inform on specific, albeit rarer, risks that are known to exist.

Self-Monitoring, Self-Quarantine, or Mandatory Quarantine?

The arrival of infected people via airplane flying from West African countries (via Europe) was made apparent by the diagnosis of Dr. Craig Spencer, who developed symptoms the day after spending the night on the town eating dinner in a meatball restaurant, riding the subway, and going bowling. Dr. Spencer was self-monitoring, did not go to work, and yet violated any reasonable definition of quarantine. Another medical professional, Dr. Nancy Snyderman, while also on a self-monitoring regime after returning from covering the Ebola outbreak in West Africa and a crew member was found to be positive for *Ebolavirus*, apparently violated that quarantine. Dr. Snyderman recently issued an apology for her actions:

> *I'm very sorry for not only scaring my community and the country, but adding to the confusion of terms that I think came as fast and furious as the news about Ebola did.*

There is no doubt that each of the violations increased the risk of infection of other people. One nurse infected with *Ebolavirus* during her treatment of Thomas Eric Duncan violated the "controlled movement" guidance of self-quarantine and traveled via mass transit. Afterward, in a news interview, she said that she would never put people in harm's way and, notably, she said: "That wasn't me." However, the mandatory quarantine is seen by some, due to mathematical models of the rate of spread of Ebola from Western Africa to other countries, as a factor that may make it less likely for health care workers to travel to Africa to help get the Ebola outbreak under control. Let's look at the statements:

> *"We do not want to put them in a position where it makes it very, very uncomfortable for them to even volunteer,"* said Dr. Anthony Fauci on *Fox News Sunday*.

But is this policy based on science, or is it based on the need to insure that health care workers go to West African countries and help end the epidemic there? While *Ebolavirus* was spreading in the US, we were reminded repeatedly by officials that policy should be based on scientific data. There is no scientific evidence that doctors, when faced with the inconvenience of mandatory quarantine, will not answer the call to help in Western Africa. When asked by

Matt Lauer on *NBC's* Today Show whether she would return after her experiences in New Jersey and Maine, nurse Kari Hickok replied with an unequivocal: *"Absolutely."*

There is, however, clear data that indicates that people under self-quarantine will, in fact, violate their quarantine. First, the observational data indicate of the health care workers and others in the US who were trusted with their own self-monitoring and quarantine violated their conditions. If an infected person develops symptoms at any time during their violation, they could easily transmit the virus to the public. Second, the Rao *et al.* (2009) study supports concerns that a surprisingly large number of people trusted with their own quarantine might willfully place others at risk of infection. Whatever the individual reasons each person may have for willfully putting others at risk, this aspect of human behavior has to be factored in any consideration of whether people should be left to their sense of responsibility to society with a scourge as deadly as EVD. Federal law in the US allows prosecution for violation of quarantine (Appendix 1).

Samantha Power, the US ambassador to the United Nations, told *NBC Sunday* news show "Meet the Press":

> *We need to encourage more; we need many more than are going right now. And we need to find a way when they come home that they are treated like conquering heroes and not stigmatized for the tremendous work that they have done.*

(10/26/2014)

Others feel that potentially exposed health care workers to others could lead to transmission, and that this should not be ignored. It is fair to wonder if the same level of evidence required of drug trials was applied to policies that could unleash hundreds of cases of EVD upon the American public.

In addition, anyone who would want to eschew keeping company with anyone potentially infected with *Ebolavirus* could not be accused of "stigmatizing" them for whatever they did that caused them to become infected. It is a large leap of logic to say that people will stigmatize doctors for trying to save lives. I think most Americans would only judge or stigmatize health care workers not for trying to save lives, but for their actions, decisions, and behaviors upon returning to the US. Most Americans would have a negative reaction to anyone whose actions put others in harm's way, intentionally or otherwise.

The statements on the expected behavior of health care workers, if isolation were to be enforced, are irrational; they are founded in fear, and the assumption that the workers would not want to return to Africa. This is really are a matter of opinion. The health care workers sacrifice their time, and take risks, and if anything, the public would react with increased appreciation for them enduring such a sacrifice. At the same time, removing health care workers from medical service for three or more weeks could have a prolonging effect on the epidemic. However, the US Government could also establish very posh quarantine conditions, within which those quarantines could be seen as a paid vacation-type reward for the effort. Members of the military see their quarantine time as paid vacation. Moreover, the most important determining factor here is the "spin" put on this by these government officials. While they had the nation's attention, they could have stated that while quarantine may unfortunately be needed, those who endure quarantine deserve our utmost respect. They needed to do what Dr. Gavin MacGregor-Skinner reported: People in West African countries who survive EVD are treated like heroes so they do not become stigmatized. In December 2014, the US CDC and the government of Sierra Leone announced they were providing support to survivors — replacing essentials like bedding and clothing. In neighborhoods, where EVD survivors are returning, they are also providing a humane counseling program to educate neighbors on the low risk of transmission after recovery. That said, a Liberian woman was recently infected after hopes of eradication by her boyfriend weeks after his recovery from EVD. This brings aspects of policy into question. This follows a model used by a company in Liberia (Firestone Liberia) earlier in 2014. The company went to great lengths to help their community understand the need for isolation and quarantine of entire families as a means to reducing transmission (Rachael Rettner, "How a Liberian Rubber Plant Prevented Ebola Spread," *Live Science*, Oct 21, 2014). However, when people do anything that places other people at risk, according to Ken Kam, then naturally, we don't like it when that happens, and we tend to, and we should, hold them accountable. The government officials seem to think the US population is more likely to adopt a mob mentality than to perform their own, informed risk assessment analysis given the information available to them. To mislead the population and to be found out in this setting would compound fear. Perhaps we should also look to the Firestone Liberia program as a model for future outbreaks that might occur (EVD or other).

Another factor that can influence the rate of spread of EVD in Africa is the availability of personal protective gear (PPG). The CDC was criticized for suggesting that it was okay to re-use PPG after disinfection; that is still a common practice in Africa, out of necessity. Our response to the crisis, our standards, may in some ways make it harder for Western African countries. People in Africa have to use whatever they have. As a direct result of the cases of EVD in the US, hospitals across the US are buying up the supply of PPG. There are reports of shortages of PPG in countries that need it most, like Sierra Leone. As early as August, the CDC stockpiled $2.7 million worth of personal protective equipment. At that time, the number of EVD cases in Africa was around 4,000. Companies reported that they were unable to keep up with demand even then. The same mathematical concern that says that we should prioritize return of health care workers over their quarantine in the US should be applied to stockpiling supplies of PPG. Hospitals with excess equipment could arrange donations to the Red Cross, WHO, and Doctors Without Borders (Médecins Sans Frontières; MSF).

The medical community's response to the outbreak can also be seen as a grave concern for increased number of imported cases. Those on the frontline during previous outbreaks are career health care workers involved in the control of EVD. They are experienced and familiar with the protocols. As thousands of doctors and nurses respond to the urgent need for care in Africa, they are much greater in number, and they may not be as careful or skilled in self-protection. Thus, the need for urgent care in Africa also drives an increased need to prevent importation of new cases here in the US. There are hundreds of people being monitored around the US at this time; the procedures in place may work at small numbers. However, in some places, the CDC and WHO had, at times, lost track of transmission chains, and *Ebolavirus* was free to roam the population.

No Mutations?

During the first House Oversight hearings on Ebola in mid-October 2014, Dr. Thomas Frieden, director of the CDC, was asked whether there were any mutations in the strain of the *Ebolavirus* responsible for the 2014 outbreak and epidemic. He replied that he *"would be concerned if there were mutations, but that there are none."*

That was a factually inaccurate statement, and was clearly unwarranted.

In fact, the data from genome sequences from EBV patients in Africa this year showed numerous mutational difference (a.k.a. "variants"), including some that in fact lead to a change in an amino acid. Sequences differ by as much as 3%. This may not seem to be a large difference between two organisms; however, single amino acid substitutions are known to lead to very large differences in function. The genetic distance between humans and chimps is only around 1%. It would appear that this strain is, in fact, a different virus, a conclusion supported by phylogenetic analysis of the data (Baize *et al.*, 2014; Dudas and Rambaut, 2014).

More importantly, the individual amino acid differences due to the nucleotide difference can lead to changes in the protein structure, and can lead to changes in the viral biology, and thus the etiology of transmission. Whether any of these mutations are responsible biological differences in virus related to the outbreak is, as we have seen, unknown. Research is needed that is focused on the potential functional significance of variation in emerging diseases, which can, at least in principle, include recombination among related Ebola strains (Wittman, 2007).

Can Humans get Ebola from Dogs?

Consider the following statements:

There is no evidence that dogs can transmit the disease.

Dogs cannot transmit the disease.

The first may be true, but it is not equivalent to the latter statement.

There is convincing evidence demonstrating dogs can become infected by the virus. In a 2006 study undertaken in Gabon, stray dogs eating carcasses of Ebola victims were found positive for the presence of Ebola antibodies. The concerns include that dogs could be carriers of the disease, or move the virus around on the fur, paws, or nails.

The CDC currently does not recommend routine testing of dogs exposed to people with EBV. This seems risky, as there is no scientific evidence that dogs cannot carry the virus. In short, they are not erring on the side of caution.

This action implies, under the principles of "evidence-based medicine," that because there is no evidence, there is no concern and no need to be wary of dogs that may have been exposed to Ebola positive patients. Dr. Well's missive on negative evidence comes to mind.

Compare this to the following possible position, which errs on the side of caution:

It is unknown if dogs can transmit the disease. Dogs exposed to the virus should be quarantined until they no longer test positive for the virus.

The deciding point of whether the conclusion "there is no concern" is warranted depends on whether there have been studies, or observations, that indicate that dogs have served as carriers to — and have infected — humans.

The tenuous nature of this line of evidence is frustrating, because the studies have not been done. Animal studies in which saliva from infected dogs is used to infect primates or cell cultures should be conducted as soon as possible.

Policy Assessment

The risk of a widespread epidemic is consistently increased by unqualified, incorrect statements. The health care workers from any country who go to the frontlines to treat people sick from EBV are seen as heroes; their willingness to endure the 21-day quarantine needed to insure the safety of the American public could also be seen as further reason to respect them. The CDC and NIH policies appear to be aimed at being ready to treat Ebola cases as they arise in the US. This is a fairly passive, defensive and reactionary approach. While reducing the number of cases in Western Africa is key to reducing the risk of importation of EVD, primary reliance on finding cases and contact tracing fails to capitalize on opportunities to rationally prevent the arrival, incidence and transmission of *Ebolavirus* in the US population, and leaves open opportunity for eventual epidemic due to missed arrivals, direct and indirect transmissions, and the possible transfer of *Ebolavirus* from the human to the pet populations which are immense.

Conclusions

A number of policies are found to be based on unwarranted conclusions from consideration of information and knowledge. Those that require more data should fall into the "unresolved" category, and should be addressed by new scientific evidence via properly powered, controlled and peer-reviewed studies. In one case, a low overall degree of concern of an outbreak was attributed to "no mutations," when in reality, peer-reviewed studies demonstrated that mutations do exist in this strain. The stated policies, positions, guidances and recommendations appear to be biased toward accepting the null hypothesis in absence of evidence available to test the hypothesis, or worse, lack of knowledge of available, robust evidence. This type of thinking can increase the risk of the spread of infectious diseases. Certain policies (e.g., no mandatory quarantine) appear to lack any backing by scientific data and, in fact, controvert available scientific data that indicate that the risk of undesired outcomes is higher than expected. The risk of exposure of people in the US to *Ebolavirus* can only be increased by these practices.

Recommendations

The following is my best attempt at an accurate and useful summary of recommendations based on warranted statements and conclusions based on data:

"People with *Ebolavirus* in their blood without symptoms are certainly contagious under certain, perhaps unlikely, situations. The likelihood of transmission via these unlikely circumstances increases with the prevalence of the disease in the population. People with symptoms are particularly contagious, and are highly contagious near the end stages of the disease, if untreated. There have been numerous transmissions of uncertain origins. Extreme caution is warranted when approaching belongings and pets of people who eventually test positive for *Ebolaviruses*. Dogs may be reservoirs of the virus, and transmission to humans from dogs cannot be ruled out. There are genetic differences between this outbreak strain and previous strains; however it is unknown whether any of the biological differences due to these mutations affect the transmissibility of the virus. Proper hydration is essential for improving a patient's odds of survival. Treatment with plasma from survivors may have helped reverse the course of the disease in very sick patients, and should be attempted whenever possible; immunoglobulins should be stockpiled between outbreaks. Scientific data exists that indicates that a significant proportion of people, including health care workers, are likely to violate self-quarantine, and thus some penalties of some kind should exist for those who do violate isolation guidelines, for putting others at risk. Quarantine insurance options should be created for health care workers in anticipation of a pandemic. Individuals who do not violate the terms of quarantine should be rewarded with merit pay.

"Studies are needed on methods designed to reduce transmission; clinics need to anticipate massive volumes of waste, much of it from vomiting and diarrhea. We need to better understand whether any of the mutations that exist enhance Ebola guinea's transmission via these symptomological changes. The FDA will now consider data from clinical studies with non-canonical designs as long as the alternative approaches involve steps to reduce bias. Doctors are encouraged to treat first, file later for compassionate use of what they determine to be promising drugs."

As Dr. Adolfo Garcia-Sastre told me:

> We need to think two things: First, we need to find the best way to stop the ongoing outbreak, and second, we need to never become complacent between outbreaks again. We need continue to work on these problems. We must be more prepared.

In my conversation with Dr. Michael Osterholm, I was left feeling confident. He said:

> Public health policies have evolved quite a bit in the last six months, and I believe that we have reached a reasonable place. Interventions are working, and case fatalities are down.

References

Baize S, Pannetier D, Oestereich L, *et al.* (2014) Emergence of Zaire Ebola virus disease in Guinea. *N Engl J Med* **371(15):** 1418–25. doi: 10.1056/NEJMoa1404505.

Bausch DG, Towner JS, Dowell SF, *et al.* (2007) Assessment of the risk of Ebola virus transmission from bodily fluids and fomites. *J Infect Dis* **196(Suppl 2):** S142–7.

Benjamin J, Li L, Patterson C, *et al.* (1996) Population and familial association between the D4 dopamine receptor gene and measures of novelty seeking. *Nat Genet* **12(1):** 81–4. doi:10.1038/ng0196-81.

Canty N, Gould J. (1995) The Hawk/Goose experiment; sources of variability. *Anim Behav* **50:** 1091–5.

CDC. (2014) Review of Human-to-Human Transmission of Ebola Virus. October 2014. [http://www.cdc.gov/vhf/ebola/transmission/human-transmission.html accessed Dec 7, 2014]

Desai R, Pannaraj PS, Agopian J, *et al.* (2011) Survival and transmission of community-associated methicillin-resistant *Staphylococcus aureus* from fomites. *Am J Infect Contr* **39(3):** 219–25. doi: 10.1016/j.ajic.2010.07.005.

Dudas G, Rambaut A. (2014) Phylogenetic Analysis of Guinea 2014 EBOV Ebolavirus Outbreak. *PLOS Current Outbreaks,* May 2, 2014, Edition 1. doi: 10.1371/currents.outbreaks.84eefe5ce43ec9dc0bf0670f7b8b417d.

Ebstein RP, Novick O, Umansky R, *et al.* (1996) Dopamine D4 receptor (D4DR) exon III polymorphism associated with the human personality trait of novelty seeking. *Nat Genet* **12(1):** 78–80. doi:10.1038/ng0196-78.

Feynman, RP. 1986. Personal Observations on Reliability of Shuttle. Report of the Presidential Commission on the Space Shuttle Challenger Accident.

Francesconi P, Yoti Z, Declich S, *et al.* (2003) Ebola hemorrhagic fever transmission and risk factors of contacts, Uganda. *Emerg Infect Dis* **9(11):** 1430–7.

LoBue V, DeLoache JS. (2008) Detecting the snake in the grass: attention to fear-relevant stimuli by adults and young children. *Psychol Sci* **19(3):** 284–9. doi: 10.1111/j.1467-9280.2008.02081.x.

Rakison DH, Derringer J. (2008) Do infants possess an evolved spider-detection mechanism? *Cognition* **107(1):** 381–93.

Rakison DH. (2009) Does women's greater fear of snakes and spiders originate in infancy? *Evol Hum Behav* **30(6):** 439–44.

Rao S, Scattolini de Gier N, Caram LB, *et al.* (2009) Adherence to self-quarantine recommendations during an outbreak of norovirus infection. *Infect Contr Hosp Epidemiol* **30(9):** 896–9. doi: 10.1086/598346.

Shaib *et al.* (2014) Ebola Virus Disease Outbreak — Nigeria, July–Septermber 2014. Morbidity and Mortality Weekly Report.

Wittmann TJ, Biek R, Hassanin A, *et al.* (2007) Isolates of *Zaire ebolavirus* from wild apes reveal genetic lineage and recombinants. *Proc Natl Acad Sci USA* **104(43):** 17123–7.

11

A Rational Analysis of Irrational Decisions, or Don't Fear the Reaper

This chapter is a final plea. People across Western Africa are losing loved ones. While initially many villagers feared that outsiders were bringing Ebola to their village, they now seem to understand and are reporting their sick, dying, and dead. People in Uganda have stopped kissing to reduce the rate of spread of *Ebolavirus*. Liberia has suspended football games. At the request of President Yoweri Museveni, the population is being more aware and limiting physical contact. Health care workers in Western African countries only elbow-bump instead of hand-shaking or high-fiving. People no longer embrace at worship. People are being told to stop touching dead bodies and, against custom, are becoming more accepting of allowing non-family members to handle burials, and the practice of cremation. Deep-seated cultural norms such as washing of the dead by a same-gendered family member are being abandoned. Because they understand now, people are being asked to change, and are changing, their behaviors, habits and ways of thinking.

Irrationality abounds in reactions due to fear. In late December 2014, a Japanese man in his 30s returned home from Sierra Leone and developed a fever. He reported touching a bag containing a person who had died from EVD without special protection. On the day he tested negative, the Nikkei index had dropped 17,628.15 points (a 1.1% loss) by midday. Health stock soared. As of this writing, this is an open story; his negative test is indeterminate until the 21 days have passed.

Given the uncertainty that exists about *Ebolavirus*, many more cultural and behavioral changes are needed. People in the US who may be infected due to their travels should not have to be asked to, but should willingly avoid contact with other people; there should be no more cases of health care workers violating their self-monitoring routines to travel on planes and on subways, as predicted by past scientific studies (Rao *et al.*, 2009). Compared to the suffering of the people in Western Africa, the minor inconvenience of three weeks or so downtime for the good of the many does not seem too much to ask. Governments should create quarantine pay for health care workers for three to four weeks so they can be kept away from hospitals until two negative tests after 21 days. There could even be merit pay for this; it's worth it.

In the last chapter, referencing how the CDC's policies with regard to isolation and quarantine are based purely on observational data, and that no trial designed to demonstrate human–human transmission could be ethically conducted, I used the following line:

> *No one should ever be subjected unnecessarily to infection with ebolavirus, or to death from EVD.*

Some think that this is precisely what the FDA is doing with the requirement of placebo-controlled trials for novel EVD treatments. The FDA seems to be adjusting their behavior slightly, and allowing translational progress with studies. But they need to go further. They need to encourage rapid trials, even those that may be underpowered — in search of results that show promise. Their concern over covariates that might confound interpretation, such as changing standards of care, are valid. However, it is not clear that the FDA applies the same standards to their own research. A study of dose effects of bisphenol A (BPA) on developing rats by FDA scientists is a good example (Delclos *et al.*, 2014; Churchwell *et al.*, 2014). The authors concluded that, while large doses had negative consequences on rat embryonic development and growth, there were no harmful effects from low doses of BPA. BPA is a substance found in many food packages and is thought to have strong hormone-like effects on developing animals. BPA is banned in baby bottles in Europe and Canada.

Critics of the FDA study point to the conclusion as not substantiated due to, among other things, the fact that BPA contamination (at low doses) was too prevalent in the environment of the study that the finding of "no effect" at low doses was not due to no effect, but rather due to the same effect as the low dose in the environment. Another flaw is that the conclusion is being used as an indication that background levels of BPA are safe, while the study did not bother to look for any neurological effects, for example, changes in learning, memory and behavior. The study may be confounding the lack of difference at low dose for the wrong reason. In spite of the fact that the original study self-identified the potential limitation of the study, the FDA has doubled down on their conclusion.

Some of the concerns about the experimental Ebola trials can be addressed by experimental design methods known as "covariate matching." The FDA is aware of these designs, but routine fails to take results from such studies seriously. Some researchers do not think they should pre-empt and short-circuit the peer review process by publishing proclamations that would restrict researchers to particular study designs. Some even feel that they should go completely in the other direction — that they should issue a blanket compassionate use approval of any and all Ebola vaccine trials for any and for all. Consider the case of Dr. Kent Brantly, who received both an immune plasma infusion from his 14-year-old former patient, and a dose of Zmapp^{TM}. Not until he received the dose of Zmapp^{TM} did he begin to show signs of recovery, but for those present, the transformation was remarkable. Anecdotal evidence with a sample size of 1, if it occurs with extreme results, is still evidence, and should be considered. I was speaking with a well-respected infectious disease researcher about this subject as the events were unfolding. Their view? "This isn't witchcraft; those drugs have been through animal trials, with great success. It's like this all the time with the FDA. There is no commitment to translation. And absolutely never, ever any sense of urgency."

There is certainly risk to individual patients if an experimental drug's safety is in question. Recall Tekmira's drug studies that revealed that a large dose could actually initiate the cytokine storm earlier in the progression of the disease. Most think the FDA overreacted by bringing the entire study to a halt (Tekmira has been issued a reprieve). However, there could also be more creative, tailored, "limited use" declarations, such as "TKM-Ebola is not to be used at high doses, or only when evidence of a cytokine storm has presented." To facilitate, the FDA could invite companies to author limited use statements in good faith, for review.

Certainly many, many people in drug and device development believe that the FDA, and their peers, should let researchers doing urgent studies state their practical study design needs, and that they should be allowed to move forward when the studies that can be done have been done. We do not have, as Ken Kam so eloquently pointed out to me in our conversation, eight years with EVD to wait for the standard rate of progress. While the logical superiority of placebo-controlled trials is clear, the ethical superiority is not clear in the context where hundreds of thousands may die. For many, even small observational studies, in which patients are given larger vs. smaller doses, would be morally superior to condemning half of the patients in a study to death. The FDA should facilitate any and all trials. People involved in the direct treatment of Ebola need data support: People to collate clinical data, including treatment, symptoms, and outcomes.

I have tried to outline a rational basis, and a utility, if you will, of fear; I have pointed out how government agency officials will cite observational data in support of policy views, and how, and why they will base policies on speculated outcomes. There is clearly a need for exigent trial design approval. And the reasons are compassion, and love. Ken's passion comes from the loss of his dad. My passion, in everything I've ever done in biomedical research, is my mom. Even Karl Popper, the father of modern hypothesis-based scientific inference, once explored the rational basis of love. If ever there was a time to ease restrictions, think creatively, to allow compassionate use, to lessen the bureaucratic burden, the time is now. With an R0 greater than 1, every sick patient guarantees (statistically) more cases. In a period of exponential spread of disease, the potential benefit of each compassionate use extends to untold many down the future transmission chains; the potential harm of side effects, to one. We should develop an Urgent Epidemic Clause on all clinical trial protocols and FDA Approval Processes, which, by direction of the director of the FDA, could unleash the full potential of good on any and all available clinical trial options. And, of course, the drug companies should be diligent in finding their matched historical controls. In some cases, the data might have existed, but was never collected. This needs to be improved, as well.

This book will hopefully serve numerous purposes: To educate a relatively complacent public about the biology, continuing dangers and stark realities of EVD; to highlight some potentially serious flaws in the customs and practices of some of the institutions charged with ensuring the public health, and to highlight what is known, but more importantly, what is not yet known about Ebola guinea. I hope to inspire new areas of research needed to better understand *Ebolavirus* in nature and in the context of human transmissions. Americans are currently ambivalent (December 2014) about the Ebola crisis. To many, it's out of the news cycle. Certain news sources such as *NPR* diligently continue to tell the stories that reflect the great truths. Specific non-governmental organizations continue to work day and night on the problem, and are making inroads. The most exceptional of these were noted recently by Dr. Margaret Chan, Director-General of the WHO Doctors Without Borders (a.k.a. MSF), Unicef, and others are making a positive difference by providing direct services. To this list I would add the Elizabeth R Griffin Research Foundation. A portion of the proceeds of the sale of this book will be donated to these organizations.

My most ardent and final plea is to the US policy makers at the CDC and the NIH, and to the politicians. Please see yourself in your own social context. Please know that the American people, and US health care workers, place an immense value and trust in your words. Please accept that in addition to telling us what is known, and sharing what is known, it is equally imperative to admit to us, and perhaps more importantly, to yourself, what is not yet known. Then tell us the work, or research, that needs to be done so the answer can be known. It is far more dangerous for our species to think that we know how to manage, control and reverse this epidemic, and future pandemics, and be incorrect, than it is to risk the troubling outcome of enabled drug companies who want to help, and concerned citizens speaking their minds, changing their habits, having three weeks' paid vacation, and acting out in response to the possibility that a large-scale epidemic could take hold in the US. We need to know what we need to know to be prepared, and a first good step in that direction would be to find out why this virus, compared to the strains from past years, is so good at transmission. Available indications are that this strain is an enteric virus that causes vomiting, not the classic hemorrhagic strain. We need to fund and do hypothesis-based science to study these very likely biological and clinical differences, so we can make changes in medical care goals and public health policy practices, and in the rendering of molecular solutions for the early detection and treatment of this Ebola guinea.

Current projections from the WHO are that Ebola should be stabilized in Africa by mid-2015. This is updated from the past projections of February 2015. Modelers state that if countries can isolate 70% of the sick and bury 70% of the dead, a steady state can be achieved. By December 1, WHO isolation goals had been met in Guinea and Liberia, but not in Sierra Leone; all three are reported to have achieved the WHO goals for safe burial. For many, the goal of steady state, and this approach, is also cruel, and is not acceptable. If we aim to contain, and we fail, we have a pandemic. We need to aim to eradicate. The mantra in terms of giving aid should be: "Too much is not enough." Even when the total number of known cases becomes very low, the risk of a resurgence is very real. While perhaps unlikely, the epidemic could return at number much larger than seen to date. Our medical priorities should be to prevent anyone from ever having symptoms that spread the virus in the first place, and to prevent anyone who has the disease from dying. We should immunize health care workers first, yes, and also those who bury the deceased, and we should create vaccine bubbles around outbreaks. But here should never, ever be any "containment centers." These centers are the concentration camps of our generation, and should serve as a meter of the global community's compassion. If they exist, it is a sign that we are failing as compassionate people to do everything we can do to bring this to a halt. We need urgently to create a device capable of detecting *Ebolavirus* in asymptomatic infected people, so their isolation and treatment can begin sooner, with lowered risk of transmission to health care workers and to other patients.

Don't Fear the Reaper

You have the gift of a brilliant internal guardian that stands ready to warn you of hazards and guide you through risky situations. You have more brain cells than there are grains of sand on your favorite beach, and you have cleverness, dexterity, and creativity — all of which powerfully combine when you are at risk — if you listen to your intuition. Only human beings can look directly at something, have all the information they need to make an accurate prediction, perhaps even momentarily make the accurate prediction, and then say that it isn't so. Denial is a save now, pay later scheme.

— Gavin de Becker, *The Gift of Fear: Survival Signals That Protect Us from Violence*

I have never been afraid to speak the truth to authority. I have suffered the consequences. Whether this trait has provided a net benefit or cost to me remains to be seen. But then, this book is not as much about me as it is about my being willing to say, and to help others say, what many have thought, and perhaps many have wanted to say. It's about the institutions and the processes that were laid bare for the public to see by the bright light of the Ebola scare of 2014. My hope is that one benefit of this crisis is the type of deep and meaningful self-examination that the modern industry of clinical science desperately needs. There are lessons here that go well beyond infectious diseases. Just because deaths due to diseases are geographically diffuse does not mean that we do not have an epidemic. Other diseases are eating away at our society for the lack of treatment options due to the same fundamental flaws in the set-up at the FDA as have been exposed by EVD. That is not to say the FDA has done no good... it is to say they need to do more good, faster. We need to reform medical research, and its foundations. We need to bring about a way of doing science where accomplishments matter more than recognition for those accomplishments. Profit is relevant, and important, but it alone should not determine which clinical options are available to the population. That seems perverse. The necessary changes begin, I believe, with a method for a truly rational analysis of policy.

One idea is to look at the way Federalism is implemented in crisis response institutions such as Department of Homeland Security and the CDC. There is a tendency these days for federal institutions in the US to assume total responsibility for every aspect of a particular flavor of crisis, regardless of local exigencies and circumstances. When the one-size-fits-all solution does not fit, the net result is a loss of public trust. Dr. Patrick Roberts, of Virginia Tech, and author of the book *Disasters and the American State: How Politicians, Bureaucrats, and the Public Prepare for the Unexpected* (Cambridge Publishers, 2013), has promoted the idea that federal agencies should look at some key aspects of the Civil Defense model in setting up more effective response agencies. The Civil Defense system enlisted local experts, volunteers, and other individuals who knew the local conditions well enough to be able to respond quickly, and effectively, to the realities of a disaster on the ground. At times, their response was merely to provide key information with regard to funding needs. At others, they were there, working with pick axe and shovel, to move mountains to prevent, reverse, or mitigate disasters. Regardless of the type of threat, a key aspect that determined the effectiveness of the response was a complete and accurate accounting of the nature of the threat for which a defense needed to be mounted. This was terribly lacking in the late summer/early autumn of 2014 when the Ebola crises taunting the shores of the US (Bogoch *et al.*, 2014). For a time, in the middle of the Ebola crisis, the modality was to discuss how it's important to use "shock" to motivate people into doing the right thing. This type of heavy-handed counter response to stoke fears and mistrust seems neither responsible, nor particularly humane. Nor does it appear necessary. Outbreaks of highly infectious and deadly diseases are likely to be the new norm (e.g., SARS, H5N1 influenza, H1N1, MERS-CoV). We need to create rational, in-place policies that address, or even harness the population's natural, healthy reactions to deadly threats, not a reactionary, irrational policy that tries to either mitigate or inflame those reactions, leading to mistrust and additional fears. And we need to continuously educate the populations between outbreaks.

In analysis of what went wrong with the Ebola crisis, some see an undue emphasis on individualistic value systems and misplaced focus on the treatment of individuals instead of public health approaches in both the government institutions of the US and in the WHO's response (Dawson, 2015). When asked why no vaccine had yet been developed, Dr. Anthony Fauci (director, NIAID) cited the lack of willingness of corporations to make investment risks where there was no market. Surely we can evolve our approach to public health beyond purely utilitarian paradigms centered on profit. What medical health professionals might consider deplorable local conditions, other see as global health injustices that result from global disparities in wealth and opportunity (Ruger, 2015). Our goal should be to progressively secure improved health care capabilities in all countries. Our innate ability to accept, even for one minute, the status quo of misery for others is a mystery to me. In the immediate short term, a proposal has been made to pool the financial risk for large-scale vaccination and treatment efforts (Erfe, 2014). Bioethical analyses have yielded similar priorities (Komesaroff and Kerridge, 2014; Dawson *et al.*, 2015). Longer term efforts that facilitate truly adequate public health infrastructure are intrinsically and instrumentally important to help ensure our collective relative safety from outbreaks, epidemics, and pandemics (Cowling and Yu, 2014; Roberts, 2014).

In the broader sense, as long as massive profits are reaped by high-ranking members of these institutions, the use of those funds cannot be meaningfully re-invested into the R&D necessary to create successes in translational research. People without the means to procure translational funds for critical new medicines and technologies that can help a minority of the unwell masses now turn to crowd-sourced funding. There are innumerable opportunities to reduce human pain and suffering in these orphaned technologies and drugs. I once proposed the creation of an Intellectual Property Share Market (Lyons-Weiler, 2009). Under this model, investors could purchase shares of good ideas, and profits from those specific good ideas would pay dividends back to the investors. It is a fairly straightforward proposal; perhaps this idea might take root someday.

Fear and Government Policy

To help with rational analysis of policy in the future, I have created a simple, model designed to help a person determine when they are likely to hold on to preconceived notions in an irrational manner. What is interesting is that irrational information, including biases and subjective preferences, can be accommodated by this rational model.

Neurologists know that the decision for a neuron to fire, or not to fire, is the direct result of the sum of the inputs of activating signals (+) and inhibiting signals (−). If the total number of signals exciting a neuron is greater than the number of inhibiting signals, the neuron will fire. If they are equal in number, or if the number of inhibiting signals is higher than the number of activating signals, it will not fire.

Let's suppose your job is to have an opinion — you are in charge of policy-making, and you want to be objective, and base policy on science. To be objective, for a given issue, you could make a list of all of reasons why you should support something important, such as the quarantine of people returning to the US after a trip to a country with an epidemic disease caused of an infectious agent. Hypothetically, your list of priorities, factors, goals, and facts in support might look something like this:

> Where X_1, X_2, X_3, X_4 and X_5 are, in no particular order
> $X_1 =$ Ensure the potential patient is properly monitored;
> $X_2 =$ Protect US citizens from immediate threats of exposure;
> $X_3 =$ Meet the expectations of state legislatures;
> $X_4 =$ Create public trust in my organization;
> $X_5 =$ Have a good reputation for making the right call.

This is a purely hypothetical list; in reality, one would also consider R0, probabilities of indirect and aerosol transmission, incubation period, etc.

Next, for these factors, each one can be adjusted, using a linear scale, to reflect one's understanding of the generally accepted understanding of their relative importance (among relevant experts), such as:

> $\alpha_1 X_1$ where $\alpha_1 = 5$
> $\alpha_2 X_2$ where $\alpha_2 = 10$
> $\alpha_3 X_3$ where $\alpha_3 = 2$
> $\alpha_4 X_4$ where $\alpha_4 = 6$
> $\alpha_5 X_5$ where $\alpha_5 = 1$.

It's important to avoid choosing experts in a biased manner because they will tend to agree with you.

The next step is to introduce your own subjective adjustment, or bias, to each factor. This factor, β_i, reflects your OWN subjective belief on the importance of each factor. Where you agree with your guesstimate of the consensus, use $\beta_i = 0$:

> $\alpha_1 X_1 - \beta_1$ where $\beta_1 = +1$
> $\alpha_2 X_2 - \beta_2$ where $\beta_2 = 0$

$\alpha_3 X_3 - \beta_3$ where $\beta_3 = -1$
$\alpha_4 X_4 - \beta_4$ where $\beta_4 = +2$
$\alpha_5 X_5 - \beta_5$ where $\beta_5 = -1.$

(25)

Next, do the same for all of the reasons to NOT support mandated quarantine as Υs:

Υ_1 = Curtailing the outbreak is Africa is more important, they might not return;
Υ_2 = Lost work issues for people in quarantine;
Υ_3 = Personal liberties and freedoms (constitutional rights);
Υ_4 = Represent the wishes of the White House;
Υ_5 = Financial cost and complexity (tractability to my organization).

As with the Xs, provide the general adjustment estimates to the Υs of your own bias:

$\alpha_{11} \Upsilon_1 - \beta_1$ where $\alpha_1 = 5$, $\beta_1 = +11$ (16)
$\alpha_{12} \Upsilon_2 - \beta_2$ where $\alpha_2 = 3$, $\beta_2 = 0$ (3)
$\alpha_{13} \Upsilon_3 - \beta_3$ where $\alpha_3 = 3$, $\beta_3 = -1$ (2)
$\alpha_{14} \Upsilon_4 - \beta_4$ where $\alpha_4 = 2$, $\beta_4 = -1$ (1)
$\alpha_{15} \Upsilon_5 - \beta_5$ where $\alpha_5 = 2$, $\beta_5 = -1$ (1).

(23)

Compare $\Sigma \alpha_i X_i - \beta_I$ and $\Sigma \alpha_i \Upsilon_i - \beta_i$.

If $\Sigma \alpha_i X_i - \beta_I > \Sigma \alpha_i \Upsilon_i - \beta_i$, consider quarantine an important option. The issue of your opinion is RESOLVED. This is the case with the example numbers I have provided.
If $\Sigma \alpha_i X_i - \beta_I < \Sigma \alpha_i \Upsilon_i - \beta_i$, consider no quarantine an important option. The issue of your opinion is RESOLVED.
If $\Sigma \alpha_i X_i - \beta_I = \Sigma \alpha_i \Upsilon_i - \beta_i$, do more research to add missing parameters and update your existing parameters. Under this outcome, the issue of your opinion is UNRESOLVED.

This model can be applied to any decision-making process. It can, above all, provide a rational framework for discussion. I expect if were to be used objectively, most experts on a topic would come to similar conclusions. An interesting, inexpensive exercise would be for multiple experts to conduct this exercise independently, and compare the results. It is important to remember that one's position on these factors may change over time depending on conditions. For example, on the issue on Cost and Tractability, this may become a much more important factor if the virus takes hold in the US, and there are multiple epidemics in major metropolitan areas. It is unfortunate that this shift in priority is very likely to occur, because our priorities for death, pain and suffering should not be parochial. We are all members of the same human family.

Individual policy makers may want to examine their own thinking in these terms, to maintain awareness of their objective reasons for their opinions on policy. It can also be useful in the objective comparison of positions on topics. Outlining the options does not take a great deal of time, or effort. Attributing proper, objective weight to the various lines of evidence may be the tough part. Also, the larger the number of factors on both sides of the equality, the more likely they will, by chance, tend to become equal if a small range of numbers are used for ranking.

Finally, please note that abject irrationality can be rationally evaluated; irrational factors would either be irrelevant factors ("because my sister has blond hair"), or woefully exaggerated β_is. Either way, for most people, either type of irrationality will usually expose a bias. The second type of irrational decision would also be made apparent when, after this procedure is applied in good faith, and the individual decides against their own constellation of factor weights and biases, but cannot explain why other than to refer back to the factors, but refuses to update the factors, weights, or bias values to align their decision-making with their considerations.

References

Bogoch II, *et al.* (2014) Assessment of the potential for international dissemination of Ebola virus via commercial air travel during the

2014 west African outbreak. *Lancet*, Oct 21, 2014. pii: S0140-6736(14)61828-6. doi: 10.1016/S0140-6736(14)61828-6.

Cowling B, Yu H. (2014) Ebola: worldwide dissemination risk and response priorities. *Lancet*, Oct 21, 2014. pii: S0140-6736(14)61895-X. doi: 10.1016/S0140-6736(14)61895-X

Churchwell MI, Camacho L, Vanlandingham MM, *et al.* (2014) Comparison of life-stage-dependent internal dosimetry for bisphenol A, ethinyl estradiol, a reference estrogen, and endogenous estradiol to test an estrogenic mode of action in Sprague Dawley rats. *Toxicol Sci* **139(1):** 4–20. doi: 10.1093/toxsci/kfu021.

Dawson AJ. (2015) Ebola: what it tells us about medical ethics. *J Med Ethics* **41(1):** 107–10. doi: 10.1136/medethics-2014-102304.

Delclos KB, Camacho L, Lewis SM, *et al.* (2014) Toxicity evaluation of bisphenol A administered by gavage to Sprague Dawley rats from gestation day 6 through postnatal day 90. *Toxicol Sci* **139(1):** 174–97. doi: 10.1093/toxsci/kfu022.

Erfe JM. (2014) Reducing Outbreaks: Using international governmental risk pools to fund research and development of infectious disease medicines and vaccines. *Yale J Biol Med* **87(4):** 473–9. eCollection 2014.

Komesaroff P, Kerridge I. (2014) Ebola, ethics, and the question of culture. *J Bioeth Inq* **11(4):** 413–4. doi: 10.1007/s11673-014-9581-9.

Lyons-Weiler J. (2009) Time for an IP Share Market? *The Scientist.* [http://www.the-scientist.com/?articles.view/articleNo/27084/title/Time-for-an-IP-Share-Market-/]

Rao S, Scattolini de Gier N, Caram LB, *et al.* (2009) Adherence to self-quarantine recommendations during an outbreak of norovirus infection. *Infect Control Hosp Epidemiol* **30(9):** 896–9. doi: 10.1086/598346

Roberts RS. (2014) The Ebola Crisis as a Crisis of Public Trust. *American Interest*, Oct 15, 2014.

Ruger JP. (2015) Good medical ethics, justice and provincial globalism. *J Med Ethics* **41(1):** 103–6. doi: 10.1136/medethics-2014-102356.

Appendix 1

42 U.S.C. United States Code, 2011 Edition Title 42 — THE PUBLIC HEALTH AND WELFARE CHAPTER 6A — PUBLIC HEALTH SERVICE SUBCHAPTER II — GENERAL POWERS AND DUTIES Part G —- Quarantine and Inspection Sec. 271 — Penalties for violation of quarantine laws.

§271. Penalties for violation of quarantine laws

(a) Penalties for persons violating quarantine laws

Any person who violates any regulation prescribed under sections 264 to 266 of this title, or any provision of section 269 of this title or any regulation prescribed thereunder, or who enters or departs from the limits of any quarantine station, ground, or anchorage in disregard of quarantine rules and regulations or without permission of the quarantine officer in charge, shall be punished by a fine of not more than $1,000 or by imprisonment for not more than one year, or both.

Appendix 2: Ebola Virus Disease (EVD) Clinical Outcomes Data Form

Location: _____ Township/State: _____

Date of Report: _____

Type of Facility: _____

Attending Physician: _____ Contact: _____

Patient Information

Age: _____ Gender: _____ Ethnicity: _____

Likely Date of Exposure: _____

EVD Outcome:

Death_____ Convalescence_____

Full Recovery_____ Other _____

Describe any family or close associate outcome history:

Medical History (Indicate Concurrent (C) or Past (P))

Diabetes _____ ||Malaria _____ ||Marburg _____ ||Cholera _____ ||Lassa Fever _____

_____ || _____ || _____ || _____ || _____

_____ || _____ || _____ || _____ || _____

_____ || _____ || _____ || _____ || _____

Symptoms:

Fever: _____ Sore Throat: _____

Aches: _____ Pains: _____

Shortness of Breath: _____ Hiccups: _____

Chest Pain: _____ Loss of Appetite: _____

Trouble swallowing: _____ Vomiting: _____

Diarrhea: _____ Exhaustion: _____

Rash: _____ Coagulopathy: _____

Anuria: _____ Convulsions: _____

Shock: _____ Stroke: _____

Other symptoms:

Progression (Fever, IgM, IgG):

Day 1 _____

Day 2 _____

Day 3 _____

Day 4 _____

Day 5 _____

Day 6 _____

Day 7 _____

Day 8 _____

Day 9 _____

Day 10 _____

Day 11 _____

Day 12 _____

Day 13 _____

Day 14 _____

Day 15 _____

Day 16 _____

Day 17 _____

Day 18 _____

Day 19 _____

Day 20 _____

Day 21 _____

Epilogue

The subtitle of this book is an admission of ignorance. We know less about EVD than we thought, but now at least we know at least some of what we would like to know.

We know more about ourselves, as well. Infectious disease and poverty go hand in hand. The solution to poverty is sustained periods of peace, education, and economic opportunity. Throughout the last 300 years, the countries and the peoples of Africa have been dealt a raw deal. I explore this in some detail in a post on LinkedIn where I pose the question: "Will the Ebola Crisis of 2014 Finally Teach the Western World the Intrinsic Value of the People of Africa?" In this essay, I describe the relationship between the chronically sad situation in various places in Africa at the feet of the colonial European empires, and show how our dehumanization of African natives came home to roost in the form of two World Wars and the genocidal practices perfected by Nazi Germany. There are lessons here to avoid hegemony.

As I write this epilogue, just before going to press, the news is both good, and bad. In human morality, there is a dichotomy of views on whether we should, and the extent to which we should, take care of those less fortunate. Clearly, countries afflicted with Ebola are sick, and need help. Their recovery from this crisis will take years. It is imperative for people who have never thought of investing in a progressive Africa to take notice: If they believe they can do good by investing, the opportunities in Western Africa look excellent. Hundreds of projects fueled by small business loans (microloans) had, before Ebola, helped foster a real sense of hope. Why not raise the standard of living in these countries with macro-investments? Why not bring western medicine in the form of a globally funded, ultra-modern western-style hospital to each and every African country who will receive it? Each one should have an infectious diseases ward, constantly on the ready to handle Lassa fever, Ebola, and other unknown pathogens. Why not make the health care industry in these countries sufficiently profitable that their talent does not migrate? Progressive liberals like myself often shudder at economic hegemony and social and economic injustice. The real lesson of Ebola guinea is that the world cannot afford to let the poorest of the poor to linger in their suffering any longer. In Ebola, we have found a selfish reason to care.

We must harness this goodwill. Going forward, the view should not be as much "doing for" as "doing with." Fair trade practices for mineral wealth and natural resources are a must. Consumers can do their part by seeking out consumables manufactured in Liberia, Guinea, and Sierra Leone. They are rare, as most of these countries' economies have been based for many decades on exploitative trade, especially in minerals and other natural resources. These, and other countries could coordinate a textile export industry, and consider creating a broad economic bloc. According to Nations Encyclopedia, Sierra Leone's manufacturing industries, which account for less than 0.5% of the GDP, include "salt, knitwear and other clothing, paint, oxygen, plastic footwear, nails, soap and cosmetics, and a wide range of furniture." Liberia manufactures clothing, art, wood carving, jewelry, and furniture. Manufacturing in Guinea is similar but has lagged in scale.

Web surfers can reach some of these products online at sites such as:

http://www.amaniafrica.org/shop-fair-trade

Progressive companies such as Liberty & Justice focus on expanding the manufacturing industry in Africa, especially in ways that employ and empower women:

http://libertyandjustice.com/

Liberty & Justice. Org
302A West 12th Street, #309
New York, NY 10014
USA
Phone: +1 (415) 889 7100

Textile and fabric companies include Sayenu Industries.
Belts made in Sierra Leone can be purchased online here:

http://www.bureh.com/#!belt-catalogue/c199a

Musical instruments made in various African countries can be purchased here:

http://www.motherlandmusic.com/

Investment firms such as OPIC can effect economic recovery by strategically investing in manufacturing in these countries. Much of the current effort is home-based, hand-made arts and crafts. In Liberia, a think tank called Game Changers Liberia is promoting economic independence via this type of industry. While one of OPIC's missions is to do no harm to the US economy, what companies abroad do with the natural resources from African countries, African countries could do themselves. Other economic moves may help as well. Partial nationalization of the wealth, such as Alaska's sharing of oil wealth with citizens, could radically alter the lives of people in these countries. This may mean bad news for multinational corporations, but the natural resources of any country should belong to the people of that country. Collective bargaining has raised the standard of living in developed nations. It is key to creating sustained recovery in least and less developed countries. If capitalism has a soul, these are the countries in which it can find it.

February, 2015

There are signs of confidence that we may have reached the tipping point in bending the curves. Projections at the end of January 2015 are that we could get to zero cases in Sierra Leone by June 2015; CDC director Tom Frieden expressed confidence that we could get to zero cases worldwide (no specified time frame). Schools in Guinea closed to slow the spread of the disease are re-opening. The number of new cases overall per week appears to be decreasing in Liberia and Sierra Leone, due to the successes in education, changes in human behavior, including spread of the news that earlier treatment leads to improved chances of survival, and the massive investments made by the countries giving aid.

However, it would be foolish to believe that we can relax and relent. There have, at the time of this writing, been over 22,000 total cases and around 9,000 deaths. The data on reporting is still incomplete, and unknown transmission chains are likely to exist, especially in isolated areas. At the end of Janurary, 2015, there were around known 50 hotspots remaining. EVD is still killing people, leaving orphans, and health care workers. This is especially true in Guinea. The virus is unrelenting in Guinea, where cultural change is slow and may be impossible. Community leaders such as Imams have been tasked with spreading information about Ebola to their community; however, the Muslim community in particular remains extremely wary of western medicine. Many in Guinea still refuse to believe that Ebola is real; they still see attempts to isolate the dead as violations of strict religious codes. While local cultures should be respected, adherence to dogma that could spread a disease as lethal as Ebola to any country should be acknowledged. Hopefully, between outbreaks, the community can have a discussion about the biology of *Ebolavirus*, with religious leaders being empowered, or required, to suspend burial requirements. Again and again with Ebola we see, from Guinea to the US, societies struggling with the ethical problem of the needs (and wants) of a few vs. the safety (and lives) of the many. This lesson has been forgotten by our advances in medicine. With over 100 cases confirmed, the US is, at the time of this writing, at high risk of an epidemic of measles because the herd immunity is lacking due to a dogmatic antivacci-nation movement. The efficacy of the measles vaccine in protecting children against terrible diseases should be reason enough for parents to insist on vaccinating their children, but the so-called "antivaxxers" (people who believe vaccines place their children at risk of developing autism) fail to consider the greater good: They put others at risk by not participating in national programs for the greater good. This perspective is far more than mere 20:20 hindsight; such occurrences of cultural and institutional amnesia are certain to recur as our society becomes more reliant and trusting in technology, and we forget to respect the awesome power of biology and Nature.

The projections made about Ebola in Africa are very sensitive to assumptions, and while it is not correct to say that they are optimistic, they cannot anticipate unforeseen events that could make the situation much worse, such as a massive outbreak in a new country, or mutations that cause the virus to become more transmissible. By all accounts, hospitals in the US are still far from ready, failing readiness drills on a regular basis. Chimerix, Inc. announced that it would end the clinical trial of drug brincidofovir in Liberia due to a lack of sufficient cases. In Guinea, MSF trials of the Japanese drug Avigan (favipiravir) are ongoing. Early, unofficial results from Avigan treatment appear to halve the mortality from 30% to 15%. A second drug produced by Tekmira — an RNA interference matched more precisely to Ebola strains from Guinea (TKM-Ebola-Guinea) — are ongoing. Phase I vaccine trials continue to show promise (Sarwar *et al.*, 2015).

Plasma trials are expected to begin in Guinea soon. At the same time, the NIH announced Phase III clinical trials of two vaccines involving up to 27,000 volunteers in Liberia. NIH Director Francis Collins has predicted that it may be difficult to find 27,000 people in Liberia at risk of contracting EVD, and has suggested that effort be moved to Sierra Leone. It would seem prudent to move the trials to Guinea or to conduct the trial in all three countries.

While large sums of money are being requisitioned for drug development and vaccines; the realization of the immense efficacy of pre-symptomatic diagnosis has not captured the imagination of those holding the strings of the largest purses. Any and every effort aimed at developing new tests, or increasing the sensitivity of existing tests for Ebola should be given priority. Early treatment is a key to good outcome, and pre-symptomatic diagnosis could provide the earliest and most effective treatment. Even if there are unusually large numbers of false positives, given such a test, secondary confirmatory tests, such as RT-PCR on tissue acquired using newer, safer splenic biospies could be used for early confirmation and differential diagnosis.

In the last week of January 2015, there were fewer than 100 new cases. This is outstanding and good news. However, even if we get to zero new cases worldwide, resurgences in Western African countries are almost a certainty. In late January 2015, after reporting 37 days of no new cases, a nurse in the Kenema district working at the IFRC Ebola treatment center died, and tested positive for EVD, according to the IFRC. To reduce the chance of resurgence, Sierra Leone is dismantling — and burning — the largest Ebola treatment center in the country. The number of new cases increased for the first time in 2015 in the last week of January: 124. The new of new cases increased again in the first week of February. In the second week of February, a large fishing section of Sierra Leone (Aberdeen) was shuttered and quarantine rules put into place five fishermen who spent time together on a boat tested positive for *Ebolavirus*. Not all new cases were from registered contacts, signifying that new and unknown transmission chains still exist.

Research on *Ebolavirus* vaccines continue; a virus like particle vaccine created by GeoVax, Inc. (Smyrna, GA) is developing a virus-like particle that causes human cells to express the GP1 protein of the strain involved in the current epidemic. They are also developing a trivalent vaccine designed to provide protection against three versions of Ebola (Zaire, Sudan and Bundibugyo). Trials like this will be difficult as the number of patients decreases.

Casualties of Ebola remain, and include thousands of orphans, and survivors are reporting lasting effects of EVD, including vision problems (specifically inflammation of the eyes) blindness, joint pain, hair and memory loss and anxiety attacks. Studies are needed to sort out the possibility of a post-Ebola syndrome because data are sparse on pre-existing conditions. Early in the epidemic, The Paul Allen Foundation has pledged at least $100 million to fight Ebola, which led, among other things, to the donation of 10,000 cell phones and satellite dishes to increase connectivity among health care workers, protective gear for doctors in Liberia. The cost of getting to zero cases is estimated at $2.5 billion. The effects of the epidemic linger on the families, communities, and economies of the effected countries. Elective and even emergency surgery is rare in Sierra Leone, where the surgeon population has been especially hard-hit, further reducing the capacity of the health care community to respond to the ordinary health care needs of the population.

Further analysis of the genomic sequence data has increased our understanding of the transmissions dynamics, to an extent. Most transmissions occurred within families, at hospitals, and at funerals. Few health care worker to patient transmission have occurred (Faye *et al.*, 2015). However, during the early months of the outbreak (up to mid-August 2014), over 38% of transmissions occurred in hospitals (Merler *et al.*, 2015). The slow-down in the rate of new transmissions is attributed to the creation of Ebola Treatment Units, to shipping household protection kits and the safe burials. Early public health intervention reduces new transmissions (Lewnard *et al.*, 2014).

There now appears to be a consensus that the clade of viruses that infected Sierra Leone has replaced two other, earlier clades. Importantly, non-compliance by only a few families appears to have been a major contributor to the prolonged low-level spread in the early spread in Sierra Leone (Faye *et al.*, 2015). This observation should have implications for enforcement policies and for educa-tion of the populations during future outbreaks: They need to know of their civic duties and the threat of self-serving behavior to tens of thousands.

Our understanding of the potential biological threat of this strain is increasing as well... It has become better understood that mutations in the Guinea strains of Ebola may threaten the accuracy of diagnostic tests and efficacy of vaccines and tests for diagnosis (Gire *et al.*, 2014; Kugelman *et al.*, 2014). This includes nucleotide substitutions, amino acid substitutions, and, potentially, mutations in short interfering RNAs (Gires *et al.*, unpublished).

A study of macaque corpses in chambers designed to mimic the hot, humid environments of West Africa have shown that live *Ebolavirus* persists least one week, if not longer, on the surface of corpses after death, and at least 10 weeks internally (Prescott *et al.*, 2015). My functional mutation hypothesis of increased transmission via increased incidence of sudden vomiting without stomach pain may have an additional potential molecular culprit. Ongoing mutational analysis by Dr. Robert A. Ricketson of Hale O'manda'o Biomedical Research has resulted in the discovery of a potential pseudo-knot formation in the RNA from long, non-coding transcribed sequences. The determination of the functions of these structures should be given high priority.

The key factors to success in shutting down an epidemic for infectious agents with no treatment or vaccine now seem clearer. Populations in areas at risk should be educated between epidemics about the realities of the infectious diseases that could appear at any time. This will work against the cultural mistrust that has led to massive spread. Infectious disease treatment units should be built at the first sign of an outbreak, and the population should be educated to bring their sick to these units and that early treatment is key to survival. A screening tool is needed for early detection, and the ideal would be pre-symptomatic detection. Rules for isolation of the exposed should be in place and the population should be made to understand the importance of their compliance as a contribution to public health. Home protection gear with clear instruction will reduce within-family transmissions. Safe burials are necessary, and all religions should be encouraged to adopt a position of responsibility for the safety of their faithful. Public health officials should build and maintain relationships with the religious leaders in every province. Health care providers should be required to participate in annual BSL4 safety drilling, complete with checklists and all-stop procedures upon protocol breaches. An emergency response power hierarchy — which is distinct and separate from the status quo hierarchy — should be established in each hospital where one person is charged with knowing the correct response to an identified risk. Experimental treatments based on scientifically sound findings should be seen as part of control and should be considered part of a rapid response. Certainly funding for research on vaccines for potentially dangerous infectious agents should be given continuous high priority in spite of the rarity of outbreaks.

Since the 1970s EVD has killed around 1/3 of the world's non-human great apes (gorillas and chimpanzees). The virus has a very high kill rate in gorillas. Perhaps trials conducted on gorillas and chimpanzees (in the wild) could benefit us, and them. A study of a VLP-based vaccine was shown to be efficacious without harmful side effects in chimpanzees (Warfield *et al.*, 2014). If this vaccination program is well funded, gorillas and chimpanzees may become less endangered; we may learn from those studies which vaccines are efficacious, and the immunity of these apes in the wild may prevent transmission to humans in the future. We should certainly become better stewards of our planet, and of each other. This may prove difficult, as it is hard to do objective science, and we cannot expect to realize fully scientific medical practice, in cultures plagued by dogma.

March, 2015

What can we Infer about Virulence and Transmissibility from Sequence Data Alone?

In March 2014, a study published in *Science* measured the amount of mutations observed between *E. guinea* sequences collected from Mali in comparison to sequences collected six, and 11 months earlier in the outbreak from West Africa. They observed 11 nucleotide substitutions, and a single amino acid substitution *within the transfer of the virus to Mali* and found that the rate of mutations during this time period (six and 11 months) was similar to the rate inferred using sequences studied previously by Gire *et al.* (2014) in the *New England Journal of Medicine*.

Because their estimate of the nucleotide substitution rate (9.6×10^{-4}) was similar to previous estimates from Western Africa (1.9×10^{-3}), they concluded that the likelihood that the strain-specific approach to diagnostics and treatment was not at risk, in contrast to concerns that had previously been stated. They also concluded that the 2014 strain was not likely more virulent, and went further to conclude that it also was not likely to be more transmissible, than *Ebolaviruses* in the past, in spite of past evidence from serial passage study in Guinea pigs that demonstrated the evolution of increased virulence after five passages from infected to uninfected animals (Dowall *et al.*, 2014).

The first conclusion may, or may not be warranted by the data; an individual mutation could dramatically alter the specificity of PCR primers, depending on local sequence characteristics. Regardless, molecular epidemiologists will advocate that we stay on top of the sequences in any given geographic location. At the time of this writing (late March, 2015), the number of new cases per week is still growing, with outbreaks in numerous, geographically diverse locations. Molecular epidemiologists will also tend to favor a multivalent, or multi-strain diagnostics, vaccines, and treatments.

There are some concerns about the media's interpretation of the Dowall *et al.* study findings:

(1) The rate of mutation, contrary to common views, is not a measure of a viral strain's virulence; i.e., a slow-evolving strain can be just as deadly to a species as a fast-evolving one. Individual mutations can be very important. There are very few amino substitutions in coding regions between influenza strains with important clinical differences (Vijaykrishna *et al.*, 2015).

(2) Dowall *et al.* address current (more recent) substitution rates (Mali, late 2014 vs. Guinea, early 2014): Policies and health care practices to date, however, have been based on our knowledge of *Zaire ebolavirus* (1995). Many more differences exist between all the sequences derived from the Guinea outbreak and past outbreaks in Central Africa than the small groups of sequences they have studied from Mali compared to earlier acquired sequences in 2014. They compared Guinea sequences to Guinea sequences and found a similar rate of molecular evolution within the current outbreak as compared to past outbreaks. That is not the evolution that

most concerns me. What concerns me is the evolution that has occurred between 1995 and 2014. The contribution of genetic differences to current virulence and transmissibility of this strain is still worthy of full investigations via functional studies. Their study should conclude that the virus may have slowed down (in Mali), but it should not conclude that this strain has not evolved, contrary to many interpretations by popular media outlets.

(3) Their specific method of analysis was different from the original analysis. Powall *et al.* assumed a "strict clock" model for rate estimations. The substitution rates are based on internal and terminal branch lengths, which have been shown to be non-independent (Lyons-Weiler and Takahashi, 1999). The estimated branch lengths in their tree are longer in the group leading to the Mali cluster, and within the Mali cluster, with less individual changes among any internal nodes among the Makona. Taxon sampling density may in part be responsible for these differences in branch length estimates; however, they seem to conclude that fewer Mali mutations exist than expected. Their own study would appear to suggest an excess of mutations in the sequences as compared to the Makona neighbors.

(4) The Dowall *et al.* (2015) study itself also only compares a few Malian ($n = 4$) to many Makona sequences. Mutations tend to accumulate in growing population such as in the months between earlier 2014 and the peak of the outbreak in October. Any specific small collection of sequences after a rapid decline will not reflect the full degree of genetic diversity present in a larger population. When nature samples a small number of individuals from a much larger population, the new population is said to have gone through a genetic bottleneck. Also, in general, random loss of variation (genetic drift) is more likely in small populations.

(5) They reported that there were only 4 non-synonymous substitutions in the earlier data. However, Gire *et al.* (2014) reported 73 non-synonymous, 108 synonymous, 70 noncoding,

and 12 frameshift mutations between the Guinea outbreak sequences as compared to Zaire from 1995.

(6)   They reported that some of them had observed substitutions in non-coding regions of the genome; this is little reassurance given the increasing likelihood that these non-coding regions may in fact encode for functional RNAs (Ricketson, pers. comm.) and such mutations may influence extremely important functional aspects of viral biological such as rates of transcript important to the virulence phenotype. An example would be polymerase "stuttering," rendering new sub-epitopes. New, immunologically important small molecular weight amino acid sequences may result (such as sGP).

(7)   They cite past literature showing that changes in the evolution of virulence is complex, and conclude that this characteristic makes changes in virulence unlikely; however, the billions of copies of the virus each represent individual evolutionary experiments, and with such immense numbers, there are an astonishingly large number of opportunities in every case of EVD for new variants to emerge that may encode for important phenotypic differences.

(8)   The authors then expand their doubt on the evolution of increased virulence to that of transmissibility in a single sentence, offering no additional data contributing to the likelihood of biological shifts in transmission routes, and mechanisms.

(9)   In spite of their conclusions, they offer a vote for erring on the side of caution, for continued molecular surveillance in case the epidemic continues.

It is difficult to make functional inferences from sequences alone; the degree of virulence of a viral strain is not merely a property of the number of genetic differences, but instead depends on the biological nature of the mutations themselves, in the context of the host, and, in our case, the host's environment. Past studies have already demonstrated the lack of correspondence between the absolute amount of molecular and phenotypic evolution (Reed and Frankham, 2001). Most succinctly, the substitution rate only addresses the question of whether a virus is undergoing a faster rate of molecular evolution, not whether a specific, important phenotype such as transmissibility or virulence has changed. For example, an extremely effective vaccine could confer protection against all but one highly virulent strain; thus, our medical responses to Ebola are part of its environment, making molecular surveillance at low numbers especially important.

In this book, I have advocated a closer look at the differences in symptomology between EVD in past outbreaks with the distribution of symptoms in the 2014 strain. Any specific mutation in a coding region, or, for that matter, non-coding could, in fact, be in part or entirely responsible for the apparent shifts in the incidence of stomach pain (which appears to have decreased); vomiting (which appears to have increased); diarrhea (which appears to have increased); and hemorrhaging (which is much less frequent in the 2014 strain). This is not to say that the mutations are known that have caused these shifts in phenotype. There is no more data in the mutational data alone to support the "three close borders" hypothesis for the scale of the epidemic than for virulence.

One cannot know the amount of phenotypic evolution unless one measures it. Rates of progression, rates of spread through a population, the symptomological spectrum, host tissue preference, and the lethality are all viral phenotypes. We really have little idea of whether any of the mutations that have been observed have caused these shifts, but we do know that we are witnesses to a new and different strain of *Ebolavirus*. Cell culture studies surveying the transcriptomic responses of various cell types to infection with the various strains of *Ebolavirus*, and animal studies designed to study the importance of the functional significance of specific mutations on the manifestation of EVD symptoms, are needed to study mechanism shifts that might explain the 2014 epidemic.

Treating Vascular Leakage

Most of the medical and pharmaceutical research to date has focused on direct attacks upon the virus: Detecting it earlier, shutting down its transmission, its replication. The final, fatal stage of EVD involves vascular leakage. Two compounds, FX06 and GX06, have been found to be both effective and safe in stopping vascular leakage in numerous conditions (Petra Wülfroth, pers. comm.). Previous findings of the potential utility of two compounds, FX06 and GX06 in the treatment of systemic shock of the type associated with fatal vascular leakage represents an important potentially new treatment direction. It is being developed by F4 Pharma (Vienna), and is a major focus of a meeting in Paris in May, 2015. In this we can see an expansion of the medical toolbox: Biorisk training, early international response, prevention (vaccines), early detection (diagnostics), early interventional treatments, and now, late-stage treatment, if all brought forward as permanent responses, all reasons for hope.

References

Dowall SD, Matthews DA, Garcia-Dorival I, *et al.* (2014) Elucidating variations in the nucleotide sequence of Ebola virus associated with increasing pathogenicity. *Genome Biol* **15(11):** 540.

Faye O, Boëlle PY, Heleze E, *et al.* (2015) Chains of transmission and control of Ebola virus disease in Conakry, Guinea, in 2014: an observational study. *Lancet Infect Dis.* Jan 22, 2015. pii: S1473-3099(14)71075-8. doi:10.1016/S1473-3099(14)71075-8.

Gire SK, Goba A, Andersen KG, *et al.* (2014) Genomic surveillance elucidates Ebola virus origin and transmission during the 2014 outbreak. *Science* **345(6202):** 1369–72. doi: 10.1126/science.1259657.

Gröger M, Pasteiner W, Ignatyev G, *et al.* (2009) Peptide Bbeta(15–42) preserves endothelial barrier function in shock. PLoS One. 2009; 4(4):e5391. doi: 10.1371/journal.pone.0005391.

Hoenen, T. D. Safronetz, A. Groseth, *et al.* (2015) Mutation rate and genotype variation of Ebola virus from Mali case sequences. Science www.sciencemag.org/content/early/2015/03/25/science.aaa5646 *Science* March 26, 2015 DOI: 10.1126/science.aaa5646

Kugelman JR, Sanchez-Lockhart M, Andersen KG, *et al.* (2014) Evaluation of the potential impact of Ebola virus genomic drift on the efficacy of sequence-based candidate therapeutics. *mBio* **6(1):** e02227-14. doi:10.1128/mBio.02227-14.

Lewnard JA, Ndeffo Mbah ML, Alfaro-Murillo JA, *et al.* (2014) Dynamics and control of Ebola virus transmission in Montserrado, Liberia: a mathematical modelling analysis. *Lancet Infect Dis.* **14(12):** 1189–95. doi: 10.1016/S1473-3099(14)70995-8. Epub Oct 23, 2014.

Lyons-Weiler J, Takahashi K. (1999) Branch length heterogeneity leads to nonindependent branch length estimates and can decrease the efficiency of methods of phylogenetic inference. *J Mol Evol* **49(3):** 392–405.

Merler S, Ajelli M, Fumanelli L, *et al.* (2014) Spatiotemporal spread of the 2014 outbreak of Ebola virus disease in Liberia and the effectiveness of non-pharmaceutical interventions: a computational modelling analysis. *Lancet Infect Dis.* Jan 6, 2015. pii: S1473-3099(14) 71074-6. doi: 10.1016/S1473-3099(14)71074-6.

Prescott, J, T Bushmaker, R Fischer, *et al.* (2015) Postmortem stability of Ebola virus. *Emerg Infect Dis* **21:(5)** — May 2015. [http://wwwnc.cdc.gov/eid/article/21/5/15-0041_article accessed 2/14/2015].

Reed DH, Frankham R. (2001). How closely correlated are molecular and quantitative measures of genetic variation? A meta-analysis. *Evolution* **55(6)**: 1095–103.

Sarwar UN, Costner P, Enama ME, *et al.*, VRC 206 Study Team. (2015) Safety and immunogenicity of DNA vaccines encoding ebolavirus and marburgvirus wild-type glycoproteins in a phase I clinical trial. *J Infect Dis.* **211(4):** 549–57. doi: 10.1093/infdis/jiu511.

Vijaykrishna D, Holmes EC, Joseph U. (2015) The contrasting phylodynamics of human influenza B viruses. Elife. 2015 Jan 16;4:e05055. doi: 10.7554/eLife.05055. http://elifesciences.org/content/elife/4/e05055.full.pdf

Warfield KL, Goetzmann JE, Biggins JE, *et al.* (2014) Vaccinating captive chimpanzees to save wild chimpanzees. *Proc Natl Acad Sci USA.* **111(24):** 8873–6. doi: 10.1073/pnas.1316902111. Epub May 27, 2014.

Index